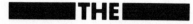

THE
Natural Healing and Nutrition

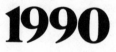

ANNUAL

1990

Edited by Mark Bricklin, Editor
and Sharon Stocker Ferguson, Associate Editor
Prevention Magazine

Written by the Staff of Rodale Press

RODALE

Rodale Press, Emmaus, Pennsylvania

The following article was adapted from and reprinted by permission of *Medical Self-Care Magazine,* P.O. Box 1000, Pt. Reyes, CA 94956 (free sample magazine available on request): "Garlic Cloves Are Treasure Troves" ("Glorious Garlic: The Science and Lore of the World's Most Popular Medicinal Herb," November–December 1988).
"What It Means to Follow Your Dreams" was adapted from *Take This Job and Love It,* by Dennis T. Jaffe and Cynthia D. Scott (Englewood Cliffs, N.J.: Prentice Hall, 1988). Reprinted by permission of the publisher.
"Update on TMJ" was adapted from *The TMJ Book,* by Andrew S. Kaplan and Gray Williams, Jr. (New York: Pharos Books, 1988). Reprinted by permission of the publisher.

Prevention is a registered trademark of Rodale Press, Inc.

Printed in the United States of America

If you have any questions or comments concerning this book, please write:
Rodale Press
Book Reader Service
33 East Minor Street
Emmaus, PA 18098

ISBN   0–87857–870–6   hardcover

Distributed in the book trade by St. Martin's Press

2 4 6 8 10 9 7 5 3 1   hardcover

Contributors to
The Natural Healing and Nutrition Annual

Writers: *Pam Boyer, Jan Bresnick, John Feltman, Mark Golin, Deborah Grandinetti, Steve Lally, Gale Maleskey, Mike McGrath, Joe Mullich, Nelson Pena, Cathy Perlmutter, Carol Piszczek, Andrew Roblin, Maggie Spilner, Melanie Stevens, Lewis Vaughn, Jennifer Whitlock, Susan Zarrow*
Production Editor: *Jane Sherman*
Designers: *Glen Burris, Peter A. Chiarelli*
Cover Design: *Darlene Schneck*
Copy Editor: *Nancy King-Bennink*
Executive Editor, *Prevention* Magazine: Emrika Padus
Associate Research Chief, *Prevention* Magazine: *Pam Boyer*
Office Manager: *Roberta Mulliner*
Office Personnel: *Eve Buchay, Karen Earl-Braymer*

Contents

Supplements and Common Sense xiii

Notice xiv

Introduction

A Practical Perspective on New Health
Answers xv

Nutrition and Health Newsfront

Snake Venom Dissolves Deadly Blood Clots 1

Oils May Tame Arthritis 2

Low B$_{12}$ Can Zap Your Zest 3

Thicken Your Bones with Walking 4

Massage Helps Mind and Body 5

Exercise Blocks the Blues 6

Sleep on Your Back and Save Your Teeth 7

Lung Precancers Slowed with B Vitamins 8

Aerobics for Asthmatics 9

Is Your Diet Keeping You Awake Nights? 10

Best Rebound Tactics for Muscle Strains 11

**Weak Link between Alcohol and Breast
Cancer** 12

Senior Swimming Is Sexy 13

Diabetics: Switch to Monos 14

Extra Weight May Cause Arthritis 15

Vitamin C to Your Teeth's Rescue 16

Eat Fish and Breathe Easy 17

Mother's Vitamins May Help Baby 18

More Exercise, Less Cancer 19

Say Hello to HDL, the Good Cholesterol 20

Vitamin E for Better Workouts 21

Recharge
Your Day-to-Day Nutrition

"Roughage" Comes of Age
From hemorrhoids to high cholesterol: Cure it with
fiber 22

Diet Profiles: Little Changes, Big Benefits
Are you eating for better or worse? Compare yourself
with these five folks and find out! 29

Mind Your Monos, Help Your Heart
A special kind of fat seems to zap "bad" cholesterol
and boost the good stuff 36

Protein: Cut Down on Beefing Up
Previously recommended amounts can make you fat
and tax your kidneys 41

Top Food Picks from the Nutrition Pros
Fat, fiber, fish oil, fruit: Find out what food scientists
feed their families 44

The Newest News on Omega-3's
Find out what's so good about fish and why you
should up your intake 49

Diet Strategies That Heal

50 Top Cancer-Fighting Foods
Tips on what to eat and how to prepare it to ward off
the big C 54

The Heart-Saver Diet Plan
This healing combo can cut your cholesterol 30 points
in 30 days 62

Fighting Fire with Oil
Arthritics beware: The oil you eat can either ease
or aggravate painful joints 69

Garlic Cloves Are Treasure Troves
A review of the scientific evidence confirming this
herb's rich healing history 72

What to Eat to Get Well Soon
Sometimes nothing is the best choice 75

The Eight-Week Lower-Your-Blood-Pressure Plan
Lifestyle changes you can make to taper down (or get
off!) the drugs 77

Beat Breast Cancer with Low-Fat Fare
Japanese women have half the incidence of American
women—and eat half the fat 87

Weight-Loss Updates

Gear Up Your Mind and Get Thin
"*You're* not the problem!" and other slenderizing
realizations 94

The Key to Big-Time Weight Loss
You need to eat a certain amount just to keep your
metabolism revving 97

Put One Foot in Front of the Other— And Leave the Pounds Behind
Motivational techniques to help you stick with your weight-loss walks 105

Tips to Lose By
Ways to quash your appetite, from the New England Deaconess Hospital in Boston................................. 107

The Diet for Diehard Snackers
Eat six meals a day and lose weight 110

Curb Your Cravings for Fat
More than anything else we put in our mouth, fat makes us fat 119

Super-Nutrient Frontiers

Why You May Need More Iron
Even mild anemia is an advanced symptom of deficiency 122

On the Verge of Cancer Breakthroughs
Updates on where research stands now—and where it hopes to be heading 127

Boron for Bones
In one study, this trace element doubled bone-maintaining hormones in postmenopausal women. 133

Counteracting Cataracts, Cancer, and More with Vitamin E
An update on the nutrient that helps cells "communicate" and organize a battle against disease 135

Head Off Heart Trouble with Magnesium
Lack of this mineral contributes to skipped heartbeats,
plaque-clogged arteries, even high blood pressure....... 143

New Roles for Protein Building Blocks
Amino acids are successfully combating severe
depression, muscle atrophy, and Lou Gehrig's
disease... 149

Big News about B$_6$
One dozen eye-opening facts about this fascinating
vitamin.. 153

Protecting and Restoring Your Good Health

Folk Cures on the Medical Frontier
Migraines, cancer, diabetes, malaria—all may benefit
from natural medicines... 159

Five Bone-Building Strategies
Why avoiding soft drinks can keep your bones hard,
and other tips... 162

Push Your Pressure Down
You don't necessarily need drugs to beat
hypertension... 165

Power Living for Prime-Timers
Succumbing to an "aging" mentality wreaks more
havoc on the body than time itself 173

Clear Up Indoor Air Pollution
Even the nonallergic can suffer severe headaches and
fatigue from mold and other nasties......................... 190

AIDS Update: What to Quit Worrying About
Many forms of contact and interaction are entirely
harmless.. 197

Bouncing Back from a Stay in the Hospital
Walking rates as the best exercise for speeding your
way to recovery 203

The Ins and Outs of Insomnia
Going a few days without sleep may make you feel
awful —but it won't affect your performance............. 205

How to Ask Smokers "Not to"—Nicely
The line between diplomatic and obnoxious can make
or break your success... 210

Cholesterol Q & A
Cookies, crackers, and peanut butter may not be as
bad as you thought 216

Eye Exercises for Better Vision
Hot controversy rages around whether or not "vision
therapy" really works 222

The Healing Power of Walking

Giving Your Ticker a Tune-Up
Keep your heart purring smoothly with regular
walking workouts 228

Get in Step with Someone You Love
Whether you're sharing your dreams or a peaceful
silence, walking can enhance intimacy..................... 231

Easing the Aches and Pains of Arthritis
Even walking only a block or two can start you on the
road to relief... 233

Slow and Steady Wins the Race
A walking program—at any pace—lets you eat more
yet stay trim.. 235

The Practical Psychology of Positive Living

What It Means to Follow Your Dreams
Most people get "practical" and give up before they
ever give their dreams a shot at becoming reality........ 241

Nip Tension in the Bud
The next best thing to eliminating the source of stress
is reducing the tension that follows 248

Jog Your Memory
Your mind needs stimulation to stay sharp just as your
heart needs aerobic exercise to stay strong................ 252

Beyond Book Learning
A host of tips guaranteed to boost your brainpower, if
not your math score... 256

Patient, Heal Thyself
We may one day be able to beat illness by
"conditioning" disease-fighting responses in
our body... 259

Body-Care Updates

Fighting Back against Backache
A guide to the best and the worst pain-preventing
exercises 264

Seven Common Causes of Contact Allergy
Here's your guide to stopping the itching and rashes ... 267

Update on TMJ
Self-help steps you can take now to relieve—or
prevent—the agonizing pain 270

How to Have Smooth, Supple Skin
Slapping on any old lotion isn't good enough—you
could cause pimples, itches, and more 279

What to Do When You Overdo Fitness Fun
Expert advice from the American Academy of Family
Physicians... 282

Chase Away the Chills
The single best piece of clothing you can wear to
warm your hands and feet is a hat............................. 293

Cater to Your Stomach's Quirks
Smart tips for avoiding intestinal discomfort, from the
American Digestive Disease Society 299

Filling Out without Fattening Up
Good news for the underweight: You only need
100 to 200 extra calories a day and a little exercise to
sculpt a new, muscular body.................................... 305

The Fine Art of Face Washing
Overzealous scrubbing and half-hearted rinsing are
two big no-nos 307

Index.. 311

SUPPLEMENTS AND COMMON SENSE

Some of the reports in this book give accounts of the professional use of nutritional supplements. While food supplements are in general quite safe, some can be harmful if taken in very large amounts. Be especially careful not to take more than these commonsense limits:

Vitamin A	2,000 I.U.
Vitamin B_6	50 mg.
Vitamin D	400 I.U.
Selenium	100 mcg.

NOTICE

The information and ideas in this book are meant to supplement the care and guidance of your physician, not to replace it. The editor cautions you not to attempt diagnosis or embark upon self-treatment of serious illness without competent professional assistance. An increasing number of physicians are ready to cooperate with clients who want to improve their diet and lifestyle; if you are under professional care or taking medication, we suggest discussing this possibility with your doctor.

Introduction: A Practical Perspective on New Health Answers

During the health craze of the 1970s, many critics assumed that the explosive interest in health would fizzle out with the pet rock. Obviously, they were wrong. What was known as the health craze then might now be called the health norm.

Not that we all exist on alfalfa sprouts and fresh carrot juice. But diehards who swore they'd never give up breakfasts of sunny-side-ups, sausage, and hash browns are now eating their hats—along with their bran muffins and fresh fruit. And most surprising to them, they're liking it and feeling great.

It's true: We're fast becoming a health-conscious nation, regularly bombarded with the newest news about nutrition and exercise. We see the latest studies reported in newspapers, magazines, and books, and on TV. Some of the information is useful. But unfortunately, a lot of it is downright confusing. Flashy headlines contradict themselves from one week to the next. Reporters give studies using 14 rats as much weight as those with 1,400 people. Well-known medical doctors passionately debate the virtues or hazards of a certain therapy, each declaring that if you don't follow his recommendation, you'll be making a serious mistake.

If all this sounds frighteningly familiar, cheer up. *The Natural Healing and Nutrition Annual* for 1990 offers a different and unique sort of health reporting. Here, we put the myriad opinions and "miraculous" discoveries into perspective for you. Chapters grow from interviews with numerous experts, giving them an authoritative base. But they also go beyond mere reporting of information, to translate scientific evidence into practical recommendations whenever possible.

These stories, then, become practical guides, helping you weave safety through the confusion with tips and hints applicable in everyday life. May you not only find them useful, but also enjoy the journey!

Sharon Stocker Ferguson
Associate Editor
Prevention Magazine

Nutrition
and Health
Newsfront

SNAKE VENOM DISSOLVES DEADLY BLOOD CLOTS

Doctors have sometimes used ancrod, an ingredient in the venom of Malayan pit vipers, to treat heart attacks.

They're at it again—this time using ancrod to help stroke patients. Small studies suggest that ancrod may, if injected within 6 hours of the event, prevent damage done by ischemic strokes, those caused by blocked blood vessels in the brain. Researchers in San Antonio, Texas; Cincinnati, Ohio; Charleston, South Carolina; and Allentown, Pennsylvania, are conducting larger human tests in hopes of eventually gaining Food and Drug Administration approval for the drug.

The venom comes from a captive colony of 400 Malayan pit vipers in Heidelberg, West Germany. Snake handlers milk them by pressing the snakes' upper jaws against the top of a glass beaker, prompting venom to drip from the snakes' fangs.

Snake venom came under study because of its anticoagulant effects, which are deadly when the venom is administered in a large dose by a Malayan pit viper. When ancrod is administered in smaller, precise doses by a doctor, the drug may safely dissolve clots in blocked blood vessels.

OILS MAY TAME ARTHRITIS

Evening primrose oil (of dubious distinction in treating premenstrual syndrome) and fish oil (of heart-health fame) may hold promise for people with rheumatoid arthritis. In a study from the Centre for Rheumatic Diseases at the Royal Infirmary in Glasgow, Scotland, 49 people with rheumatoid arthritis were divided into three groups: One received evening primrose oil, the second was given primrose oil with fish oil, and the third received an inactive oil (a placebo).

The medications were administered daily for a year. Then all three of the groups received a placebo for an additional three months. The volunteers were monitored continually for symptoms of stiffness and joint pain, and for grip strength.

The results? Over 90 percent of those receiving the evening primrose oil, with and without the fish oil, reported big improvements in these areas—and most relapsed while on the placebo. Thirty percent of the placebo group also reported a decrease in symptoms. About half of those relapsed during the additional three-month period (*Annals of the Rheumatic Diseases*).

Although these results are far from conclusive, Robert Zurier, M.D., professor of medicine and chief of rheumatology at the University of Pennsylvania, says that both fish oil and evening primrose oil contain fatty acids that, in studies on animals and human cells in culture, have been shown to suppress the production of biochemicals that cause inflammation. More research may confirm that theory.

LOW B$_{12}$
CAN ZAP YOUR ZEST

Vitamin B$_{12}$ deficiency can lead to a litany of sad symptoms: memory loss, confusion, depression, loss of balance, impotence. What's worse is that the deficiency is still often overlooked.

One reason is that many doctors test for B$_{12}$ deficiency only when a patient has a blood disorder, such as anemia, say scientists at the University of Colorado Health Sciences Center in Denver and Columbia University in New York City. But the researchers found that patients can have neurological or psychiatric symptoms caused by B$_{12}$ deficiency with no accompanying blood disorders (*New England Journal of Medicine*).

"B$_{12}$ blood levels should always be measured when unexplained dementia is present," says University of Colorado researcher Robert Allen, M.D. "Low and low-but-normal levels should be confirmed with new tests to measure B$_{12}$ byproducts, methylmalonic acid and homocysteine."

Since B$_{12}$ deficiency is usually caused by malabsorption, not low intake, monthly injections are prescribed. It may take as long as a year for mental symptoms to disappear completely, Dr. Allen says.

THICKEN YOUR BONES WITH WALKING

While scientists debate the benefits of taking calcium versus estrogen to halt postmenopausal bone thinning, Tufts University researchers are touting another preventive approach: walking.

In a new study from the USDA Human Nutrition Research Lab at Tufts, nine postmenopausal women walked briskly 45 minutes a day, four days a week, for a year. For eight months of that time, they wore 8-pound waist weights while walking. (These were primarily to build stamina, not bone mass.) The density of bones in the lower spine was measured at the beginning and end of the year.

At year's end, the walking women showed about a 3 percent increase in bone density. An inactive group of women of similar age and fitness had an average bone loss of 10 percent during the year (*Federation Proceedings*).

"From what we see, exercise may be one of the best ways to help stop or prevent age-related bone loss," says William Evans, Ph.D., chief of the USDA-Tufts Physiology Laboratory. He recommends the same amount of exercise used in the study, with or without weights. "It may not be the minimum required for bone benefits, but it's an amount we know works."

MASSAGE HELPS
MIND AND BODY

What could be nicer than snuggling up with a soft, sweet-smelling baby? Or healthier for the baby?

In a study from the University of Miami Medical School, premature babies who were caressed and massaged for 15 minutes three times a day for ten days gained weight 47 percent faster than other preemies left alone in incubators. Both groups received the same routine stimulation, such as holding and rocking.

"The massaged infants showed signs of faster neurological development and became more active and responsive than the other babies," says University of Miami Medical School psychologist Tiffany Field, Ph.D. No one knows why this happens, but researchers theorize that certain biochemicals released by touching—or others released in the absence of touch—may be the underlying factor. An interesting observation: Dr. Field has found that firm, slow strokes on a baby's back and legs help it relax, while light strokes on its face, belly, or feet tend to stimulate.

Further, in a review of the available research, Theodore D. Wacks, Ph.D., of Purdue University concluded that babies who are held more in the first six months of life were likely to have an advantage in mental development over babies held less.

EXERCISE BLOCKS THE BLUES

Exercise may help treat symptoms of moderate depression, psychiatrists have long said. Now we have evidence that exercise may *prevent* symptoms. Compared to women getting little recreational exercise, those getting at least moderate exercise (enough to lose weight or lower blood pressure) may cut their risk of depressive symptoms by half, a new study suggests (*American Journal of Epidemiology*).

In 1975, researchers led by Mary E. Farmer, M.D., Ph.D., of the National Institute of Mental Health, measured depressive symptoms and exercise in 1,900 people. Eight years later, Dr. Farmer's team did a follow-up evaluation.

The results linked little or no exercise with depressive symptoms in black and white men and women. But poverty hits blacks disproportionately, the researchers noted, and may be a stronger contributor to their symptoms. For white women, regardless of other risks—household income or employment status, for example—recreational exercise seemed to provide protection from depressive symptoms.

How might exercise block the blues? It increases norepinephrine, serotonin, and dopamine, all neurotransmitters (substances that transmit messages between nerves) that are thought to be low in depressed people. Regular aerobic exercise also boosts endogenous opiates, feel-good drugs produced by our brain. Another theory holds that physical fitness may be beneficial simply by raising self-esteem.

SLEEP ON YOUR BACK AND SAVE YOUR TEETH

If you suffer from night bruxism—grinding your teeth while asleep—you should note your position. Sleeping on your stomach or side may be the cause.

"These positions can put unnatural pressure on the face; the teeth grind in order to compensate," says Tom Colquitt, D.D.S., of Shreveport, Louisiana, a leading bruxism researcher. (Stress is considered the other main cause of bruxism.)

To stop the grinding and prevent the excessive tooth wear it causes, dentists suggest you try sleeping on your back, since this position puts the least strain on the mouth. John C. Brown, D.D.S., president of the Academy of General Dentistry, believes most people can adapt to the new position in three to four nights.

If you must sleep on your side, try placing a contoured foam pillow under your face and another pillow under your free arm. This will reduce strain on the neck and jaw and prevent you from rolling into a bad position.

If you suspect you have a bruxism problem but aren't sure, check with your dentist. He or she can check for abnormal tooth wear. Or, if problems persist, have someone watch you when you sleep to detect grinding.

LUNG PRECANCERS SLOWED WITH B VITAMINS

It's known that smokers have lower blood levels of the B vitamins folate and B_{12}. Tobacco smoke may deplete these vitamins in the cells lining the lungs. Since folate is needed for normal cell division, it's thought that a deficiency could lead to abnormal cell changes in the lungs.

That line of thinking has led researchers at the University of Alabama at Birmingham to look at both these nutrients for the role they may play in preventing lung cancer. They studied 73 long-time smokers, all with precancerous cell changes in lung secretions. About half received 10 milligrams of folate and 500 micrograms of B_{12} daily. The other half got blank pills (placebos).

After four months, lung fluids were checked again. The results? The lung fluids of the men getting the vitamins now had less severe precancerous changes.

Researchers caution, however, that this doesn't mean smokers can safely puff away as long as they take vitamins. Good nutrition may help people at risk for cancer, but it's far better to reduce the risk by quitting smoking. Further study should clarify any possible cancer-preventing role of B complex and other vitamins.

AEROBICS
FOR ASTHMATICS

People with asthma often find that physical activity leaves them winded, so they simply don't work out. In fact, working out may improve lung power and, with time, ease breathing. That's the finding of Francois Haas, Ph.D., who directs the pulmonary function laboratory at New York University Medical Center. Dr. Haas has helped people with asthma find new lives as athletes. His book, *The Essential Asthma Book,* details his exercise program.

"You should be under a doctor's care and your asthma should be stable," Dr. Haas says. Keep an inhaler on hand, and, if necessary, premedicate with albuterol or cromolyn sodium or both, 15 to 30 minutes before you begin exercising.

Try walking. Warm up first with slow walking or light stretches, then gradually step up your pace and distance. In cold or dry air, keep a scarf or mask over your mouth and nose to heat air first. Cool down with light exercise.

If attacks still occur during exercise, switch activities. Instead of walking, try swimming, Dr. Haas suggests.

IS YOUR DIET KEEPING YOU AWAKE NIGHTS?

Researchers have long known that copper and iron deficiencies can make you sluggish and fuzzy-headed. Both minerals are used to produce neurotransmitters, the brain's chemical messengers. Now a new study is the first to suggest another effect: Diets low in copper or iron may interfere with a good night's sleep.

For three months, researchers at the U.S. Department of Agriculture in Grand Forks, North Dakota, gave 11 women meals containing less than one-third the Recommended Dietary Allowance (RDA) of copper. They gave another 13 women meals with less than one-third the RDA of iron. They studied both groups for three months on normal diets.

Self-reports of symptoms showed clear patterns. While on the deficiency diets, both groups reported they slept poorly, although in different ways.

Those on the low-copper diet said that they went to bed earlier and slept longer yet felt worse when they awoke— compared to their experience on a normal diet. Those eating too little iron also slept longer but woke more often during the night (*Federation Proceedings*).

"These low levels of intake aren't that unusual in a typical diet," says James Penland, Ph.D., the study's chief investigator. "If you're having trouble sleeping, I'd first look at the most likely causes—stress, illness, medications, coffee, or alcohol. If these factors are ruled out, I think it would be more than reasonable to have your doctor check your trace mineral status."

BEST REBOUND TACTICS FOR MUSCLE STRAINS

Letting pain be your guide could lead you astray when it comes to muscle strains or tears. At a certain point in the healing process, you'd be best advised to bite the bullet and work through the pain, new research suggests.

"People assume that pain is a warning signal. But that's true only sometimes," says Wilbert Fordyce, Ph.D., a psychologist at the University of Washington's Pain Center in Seattle. "The best way to make a muscle-tissue injury better is to use the muscle. If you rest too long, your muscles will shorten and stiffen."

Generally, the rest phase shouldn't last longer than ten days for minor muscle strain; a week for upper back, shoulder, or neck strain; two weeks for lower back strain; two to eight weeks for lower back strain with complications (such as a herniated disk); or three to four weeks for a torn muscle.

After that time, people recover more quickly if they get clear instructions from their doctor for slowly reactivating their muscles. This should include exercises to be performed according to a set number of repetitions, not pain tolerance, Dr. Fordyce says (*American Psychologist*).

WEAK LINK BETWEEN ALCOHOL AND BREAST CANCER

Due to a 1987 study by Harvard University researchers, women were warned that even a few drinks a week could increase their chances of developing breast cancer. More recently, however, other Harvard researchers did an overview analysis of many of the previous studies on alcohol and breast cancer. While they did find that the more a woman drinks, the greater her risk, they concluded that for the average woman who drinks moderately (one drink or less a day), that risk is so small there's no need to stop drinking.

"It's true studies have found a link between drinking and breast cancer, but it's a very weak link," says Ernst Wynder, M.D., a leading cancer researcher and president of the American Health Foundation. In a large-scale study, he and fellow researcher Randall E. Harris, M.D., found no compelling evidence of such a connection (*Journal of the American Medical Association*).

It's important, Dr. Wynder says, to distinguish between a "link" and a "cause." "Although the two have been linked, there's no proof alcohol causes breast cancer," he says. Other factors could be involved.

Meanwhile, what are physicians and other health professionals telling their patients? Of five of the country's top cancer specialists polled (at Johns Hopkins Oncology Center, the Mayo Clinic, Columbia University's Comprehensive Cancer Center, the National Cancer Institute, and the Guttman Breast Diagnostic Institute), none said they told their patients to stop drinking to prevent breast cancer. But all said it's a good idea to drink in moderation, if at all.

SENIOR SWIMMING IS SEXY

George Burns isn't the only oldster with an enviable sex life, it seems. There are plenty out there, apparently all hanging out at the pool.

Researchers at Bentley College in Waltham, Massachusetts, surveyed 160 people ages 40 to 80—all of them active in Masters swimming competitions—about their interest and participation in sex. "We found that these men and women have sex lives more like people in their late twenties or early thirties," says Phillip Whitten, Ph.D., the study's coauthor. According to the swimmers' responses, sexual activity was 7.1 times a month for those in their forties and 6.7 times a month for those 60 and older.

Whether exercise alone produced these results or indeed, whether these swimmers' egos were more active than their evenings, could not be determined from this survey.

"The most important factor here may well be psychological," Dr. Whitten admits. "These people were proud of their bodies and they felt younger."

DIABETICS: SWITCH TO MONOS

A new preliminary study hints that monounsaturated fats may be a true friend to type II (non-insulin-dependent) diabetics, who have higher glucose (blood sugar) and heart disease risks than most people. Scientists at the University of Texas Southwestern Medical Center, Dallas, compared a low-fat, high-carbohdyrate diet—standard for type II diabetics—to a lower-carb, higher-mono (olive oil) diet. For four weeks, ten type II diabetics followed each diet.

The results were surprising. "Glucose levels were actually lower on the mono diet," says the study's leader, Abhimanyu Garg, M.D. Each diet lowered total cholesterol and LDL (low-density lipoprotein) cholesterol. The monounsaturated-fat diet, though, also lowered triglycerides and VLDL (very-low-density lipoprotein) cholesterol, thought by some scientists to be risks for heart disease, and raised HDL (high-density lipoprotein) the heart-protective cholesterol, more.

For now, most type II diabetics should stick with the American Diabetes Association (ADA) guideline to keep total fat less than 30 percent of calories. "But, if I saw a patient on the ADA diet with high triglycerides and low HDL, I'd try a high-mono diet," Dr. Garg says.

EXTRA WEIGHT MAY CAUSE ARTHRITIS

Doctors have long noted a link between obesity and osteoarthritis, but they weren't sure which came first. Now two studies have produced the first clear evidence that excess weight may cause the condition. The studies are doubly important because weight is one of only two known risk factors for osteoarthritis that can be controlled. (The other factor is injury; age and sex are "uncontrollable" factors.)

In one study, researchers from Boston University examined 1,420 participants in the famed Framingham Heart Study. They determined that people who were obese some 36 years ago, when the study began, were later more likely to develop osteoarthritis than slim individuals. The heaviest 20 percent of the women, for example, were twice as likely to develop the disease (*Annals of Internal Medicine*).

Another study of over 5,000 people, the First National Health and Nutrition Examination Survey (HANES I), had similar findings (*American Journal of Epidemiology*).

One theory is that extra weight strains the knee joints, causing arthritis. But David T. Felson, M.D., who worked on both studies, is investigating the possibility that metabolic changes induced by obesity may influence osteoarthritis. The rationale is that osteoarthritis also occurs in the hand, which should not be strained by the extra weight.

VITAMIN C
TO YOUR TEETH'S RESCUE

Taking extra vitamin C may lead to a quicker, easier recovery after tooth extractions, a preliminary study from the University of Miami suggests.

In the study, 277 patients who took vitamin C supplements (500 to 1,000 milligrams daily) for a period of one week after an extraction healed more quickly and reported less pain on average than 175 patients who received none. More important, those taking vitamin C were five times less likely to suffer the painful complication called "dry socket," an inflammation of the open socket (*Florida Scientist*). Dry socket occurs in about 1 in 20 extractions.

The researchers, Robert A. Halberstein, Ph.D., and Glenn M. Abrahmsohn, D.D.S., are now doing a 400-patient follow-up comparing the effectiveness of vitamin C versus a placebo (inactive look-alike). Early results with the first 120 patients confirm the previous findings.

The researchers also note no side effects. "This is a safe, inexpensive, over-the-counter product," says Dr. Halberstein.

EAT FISH
AND BREATHE EASY

Fish oil is suspected of having anti-inflammatory properties that may be useful in treating several conditions. Asthma may be among them, suggests a new preliminary study from Guy's Hospital in London. In the study, 15 people with asthma took 18 capsules a day of either fish oil or a placebo. After ten weeks, those taking fish oil had significantly fewer breathing difficulties in the so-called late asthma reaction than those taking placebos (*Journal of Allergy and Clinical Immunology*).

The late asthma reaction is an inflammatory condition that can come several hours after you're exposed to an allergen and have initial breathing problems. The late response is even more severe than the first reaction, so the idea of being able to mitigate it with something as simple as fish oil is exciting. Still, these results are far from conclusive and require some long-term studies to confirm them. "Right now, I tell my patients with asthma to just eat a diet with a lot of fish in it," says Mark P. Shampain, M.D., a Pennsylvania allergist who has done several studies on late asthma reaction.

MOTHER'S VITAMINS MAY HELP BABY

Women who take multivitamins regularly around the time of conception may reduce their risk of giving birth to babies with defective spines and brains. That's what a Centers for Disease Control study seems to suggest. The researchers say that the results are preliminary but are consistent with similar studies done on the subject (*Journal of the American Medical Association*).

The data were gleaned from interviews with about 3,200 mothers, a tenth of whom gave birth to babies with either spina bifida (exposed spinal cord) or anencephaly (missing brain or skull bones). Among the women who took multivitamins regularly (at least three times a week, from three months before conception through the first trimester), there was a 50 percent reduction in risk for these defects compared with women who didn't take multivitamins. An increased incidence of defects also occurred in babies born to women who took multivitamins only after conception.

No doubt more studies will follow to rule out other factors that could have been responsible for the reduced risk, such as the mother's diet. Until then, the researchers caution that women anticipating becoming pregnant should consult their doctors before taking vitamins. The head of the study, Joseph Mulinare, M.D., also reminds women that there are other important steps they can take to prevent birth defects. These include not smoking, minimizing alcohol use, using medications wisely, and getting prenatal care before becoming pregnant.

MORE EXERCISE, LESS CANCER

Being physically active has been linked to a reduced risk of colon cancer. What's more, the cancer-fighting benefit seems to increase as you become more active. So say researchers at the Utah School of Medicine, corroborating similar findings by other researchers. They reached these conclusions after interviewing 229 men and women with colon cancer about their past diet and physical activity and comparing the results to 384 carefully matched, healthy people (*American Journal of Epidemiology*).

The researchers go so far as to suggest that physical activity may even modify the harmful effects of a fatty diet, the greatest-known risk factor for colon cancer. However, Martha Slattery, Ph.D., who headed the study, cautions that this conclusion was drawn from a relatively small group. So, she says, your best bet is to exercise and eat well.

The researchers theorize that physical activity, whether at work or play, may cause food by-products and carcinogens to move through the colon more quickly. And the less time the carcinogens spend in the colon, the less damage they are likely to do. Another colon cancer expert, who calls the findings "logical, but preliminary," thinks physical activity may reduce the risk of colon cancer through an unknown, less obvious mechanism.

SAY HELLO TO HDL, THE GOOD CHOLESTEROL

You may already know that keeping your total blood cholesterol below 200 milligrams/deciliter reduces your risk of heart disease. But now evidence suggests that low amounts of HDL (high-density lipoprotein)—the "good" cholesterol—may also be a risk factor for heart disease, even if your total cholesterol is fine. The combination of insufficient HDL but acceptable total cholesterol has been linked to a greater-than-expected incidence of heart attack in a study of 2,425 men and women over age 50 by researchers in the famous Framingham Heart Study (*Arteriosclerosis*).

"We've identified a new subgroup of people at risk for heart disease who would be missed by the current cholesterol guidelines [which do not address HDL]," says Michael Miller, M.D., from Johns Hopkins University. Dr. Miller presented another study with similar HDL findings at an American Heart Association conference.

Robert D. Abbott, Ph.D., a coauthor of the Framingham study, believes that everyone over age 50 should have HDL screenings, since low levels of HDL seem to be especially risky for this age group. Some scientists say that everyone should know his or her HDL level. (HDL can be tested when blood is drawn for a total-cholesterol screening.) Researchers think that a desirable HDL level for men may be over 45, and for women, over 50. Another low-risk indicator, researchers say, is a ratio of total cholesterol to HDL of 4.5 to 1 or lower.

To raise HDL, you can lose weight (if you're obese), quit smoking, and exercise.

VITAMIN E
FOR BETTER WORKOUTS

Some athletes swear vitamin E improves their performance, even though they have little scientific evidence. Their claims may get some support, however, from a new study by German researchers. The study involved 12 high-altitude mountain climbers. During a ten-week expedition, half the group took 400 milligrams a day of vitamin E. The other half took blank look-alike pills (placebos).

Two tests were used to calculate physical performance. Muscle fatigue was measured by blood levels of lactic acid. After four weeks, the men taking vitamin E took significantly longer than those not taking E to build up to a high level of lactic acid.

The researchers also assessed cell damage by measuring a gas, pentane, that the men exhaled. (This gas is produced during lipid peroxidation, a chemical reaction accelerated by exercise that may damage cell membranes.) Four weeks into the expedition, the placebo group had large increases in breath pentane, while the E group had no more than at the start of the climb (*International Journal for Vitamin and Nutrition Research*).

What does this mean for more casual exercisers? "There is evidence that vitamin E is used up faster in exercise," says chief researcher Lester Packer, Ph.D., director of the Membrane Bioenergetics Group at the University of California, Berkeley. "More studies are needed before researchers can say that vitamin E improves athletic performance."

Recharge Your Day-to-Day Nutrition

"Roughage" Comes of Age

How should you start your day? With a big bowl of porridge! And be sure to eat lots of whole meal bread. That "veddy British" advice comes from the "fiber man" himself, British surgeon Denis Burkitt, M.D. An award-winning researcher and Fellow of the Royal Society, Dr. Burkitt, along with many notable colleagues, published influential books and articles in the 1970s linking low fiber intake in Westernized societies to the high incidence of constipation, colorectal cancer, coronary heart disease, diabetes, and other diseases.

The list of fiber's benefits is long and impressive: It can relieve constipation, may help overcome obesity, is useful in the treatment of diverticular disease and hemorrhoids, may help prevent colorectal cancer, can lower serum cholesterol levels—thereby reducing the risk of heart disease—and can play a role in the management of diabetes.

In the pre-Burkitt era, fiber was called "roughage" and was thought to "clean out the system," much as a scouring pad scrubs out a pot. The term "dietary fiber," popularized by Dr. Burkitt and his colleague Hugh Trowell, corresponds with scientists' current understanding—that fiber works within the body as an integral part of a healthy diet.

Dietary fiber is found only in plant foods—whole grains, fruits, and vegetables—and has certain identifiable traits. It absorbs water to one degree or another as it moves through the digestive system. But, unlike other dietary substances like protein, fat, and most starch, it remains undigested for much or all of the trip. It passes through the small intestine and enters the colon virtually intact.

But not all fiber is created equal. There are two main types—insoluble (which, for the most part, remains undigested) and soluble (which is eventually almost totally digested in the large intestine). Each plays a different role in your health.

Insoluble Fiber

Crunchy and crisp, insoluble fiber is found in the woody stalks, stems, peels, and skins of fruits and vegetables, and in the bran (the seed coat) of whole grains. Scientists have identified cellulose, hemicellulose (no relation), and lignin as the three plant components most loaded with insoluble fiber. They absorb water as they move through the digestive tract and stay fairly intact from start to finish—during the period that fiber experts call "transit time." The result: an increase in stool bulk and a faster journey through your system, which makes insoluble fiber a natural hedge against constipation and hemorrhoids.

Insoluble fiber has also made headlines as the type of fiber most likely to protect you against colorectal cancer. Since it's such a good bulking agent, scientists theorize that it may dilute cancer-causing substances, as well as usher them out in record time. It also may change the environment of the intestinal tract, thereby reducing the production of carcinogens, which can occur in normal digestion.

Soluble Fiber

Bite into a ripe, juicy pear. You've just tasted the kind of fiber that doesn't seem like fiber. Unlike its stalwart insoluble counterpart, soluble fiber is virtually all digested, so it lacks the valuable bulking abilities of insoluble fiber. But before it's broken down, soluble fiber forms a kind of gel as it absorbs water in the intestinal tract.

Probably because of this odd characteristic, soluble fiber tends to slow down the body's digestion of food. This means, among other things, that glucose enters the bloodstream more slowly, thus evening out sugar levels—a boon for diabetics.

And that's not all. Many studies have been conducted to test the effect of soluble fiber on both normal subjects and those with high cholesterol levels. Reviewing the results, one expert concluded that, for the most part, soluble fiber lowers LDL, or low-density lipoprotein (bad), cholesterol levels without significantly decreasing the level of HDL, or high-density lipoprotein (good), cholesterol.

The three types of soluble fiber are pectin, gums, and mucilage. Pectin, which helps to hold the plant cell wall together, is found in most vegetables, especially in onion bulbs, leeks, and asparagus shoots. Another good source is fruit, including dried fruit. You'll find it in the flesh, not the peel, of the apple or in the stringy membranes of citrus sections. Pectin's gelling abilities are well known to the makers of jellies.

Gums are found in a variety of plants. Oat bran, the star of fiber research, owes its cholesterol-lowering properties to oat gum. And, from limas to chick-peas, every legume contains its own gumlike soluble fiber. Guar gum, from the Indian cluster bean, is used to thicken or improve the consistency of prepared foods like ice cream and salad dressing.

Mucilage, a substance that keeps the plant from drying out, is found primarily in seeds.

How Much Is Enough?

Americans currently consume, on the average, between 5 and 14 grams of fiber every day. Compared to the average diets of people in many Third World countries, that's low—too low. The National Cancer Institute recommends upping the ante to between 20 and 35 grams a day.

Some experts, however, suggest that you calibrate your fiber intake according to your calorie intake. One reasonable formula: 10 to 13 grams of fiber per 1,000 calories.

Once you become familiar with fiber values, you'll discover that the best way to boost your intake is to go for the core foods, the heavy hitters in the fiber arena. And the time to get started is the morning. "Sweet buns should be prohibited by law for breakfast!" says Dr. Burkitt. "Breakfast is the best meal to get fiber because you have control of breakfast— you're at home." Wheat bran cereal is very high in insoluble fiber, while oat bran offers a 50/50 mix of insoluble and soluble (oat bran has about three times as much fiber by weight as rolled oats). But any whole grain can be counted on to make a filling, high-fiber breakfast.

Don't be shy about mixing your grains, either. Sprinkle a second, crunchier cereal over your bowl of flakes. Stir oat bran into whole grain pancake batter to add extra soluble fiber. Dried fruits and all-fruit jam provide soluble fiber as well.

At lunch or dinner, keep the fiber count rising with legumes such as kidney beans, lentils, and chick-peas. Beans are an excellent source of fiber, both soluble and insoluble, and come in enough varieties to keep your palate interested. By the simple act of adding $\frac{1}{2}$ cup of lima beans to your serving of soup, salad, or casserole, you've upped the insoluble fiber 5.6 grams and the soluble 0.9 grams, for a total boost of 6.5 grams.

Salad greens are not top fiber sources, although you can raise the fiber level by choosing your salad "fixin's" carefully. By supplementing the lettuce and tomatoes in your salad with $\frac{1}{2}$ cup of raw broccoli and one medium carrot, you add 2.2 of insoluble plus 1.5 of soluble—3.7 grams total fiber. And counting a half cup of chick-peas, you'll come away from the table 10.2 grams richer!

Clearly, fresh fruit can't match grains or beans for fiber. You'd have to eat 12 medium apples to get the amount of insoluble fiber in a cup of wheat bran cereal. But apples have something wheat bran's short on—soluble fiber.

Whenever possible, eat your fruit the way nature grew it. Choose an apple over applesauce, a whole orange instead of juice. That way you'll get both kinds of fiber, plus all the built-in nutrients.

More fiber help:

• Dessert doesn't have to be a low-fiber affair. Enjoy an apple tart or fig bar made with whole wheat flour.
• Snack on popcorn, dried fruit, or a whole wheat pita pocket warmed in the toaster oven.

● Drink plenty of liquids—fiber simply can't do its job without adequate fluid consumption.

Easy Does It

The antisocial aspect of certain high-fiber foods is all too well known. Beans, cabbage, and broccoli are common of-fenders. But it is possible to cut down on gas as well as diarrhea and bloating—common symptoms of the startup period.

● Increase your fiber intake gradually, so your system has a chance to adjust.
● If you notice that certain vegetables give you gas, eat them cooked instead of raw (cooking alters fiber's form but does not significantly decrease the fiber content).
● Chew slowly and thoroughly to reduce digestive distress. Bonus: You may end up eating less because you'll reach a feeling of fullness before your meal is finished.

If you have kidney disease, diabetes, a bowel disorder, or other serious health problems, get a doctor's go-ahead before increasing your fiber intake. Fiber can produce inflammation or abdominal distress in people whose systems are not equipped to handle it.

What about Fiber Supplements?

Eating a high-fiber diet has hidden bonuses. Fiber-packed foods really satisfy. What's more, they tend to be high in vitamins and minerals and very low in fat. So a shift to a fiber-rich diet is a shift to a more healthful diet overall. That's why experts believe that getting fiber from foods is preferable to taking fiber supplements.

Still, hectic lifestyles sometimes interfere with the best diet-wise intentions. If you find that your fiber intake consis-tently falls short of the guidelines given earlier, you may want to consider a fiber supplement. Choose the type that's made of compressed, coarse fiber, like wheat bran or soy fiber.

The ground-up husk of the psyllium seed yields a gummy fiber used to make psyllium muciloid—a bowel regulator (thanks to its insoluble fiber component) and a good source of soluble fiber. Steer clear of powdered cellulose, however. Al-

UPGRADING THE STAFF OF LIFE

Switching to a high-fiber bread is an easy way to slip more fiber into your diet.

High-Fiber Oat Bread

1 medium potato

2 tablespoons honey

1 cup whole wheat flour

1 cup unbleached flour

2½ teaspoons baking soda

1 teaspoon cream of tartar

½ teaspoon salt

¾ cup rolled oats

¼ to ½ cup currants or raisins

Coat an 8-inch round cake pan with vegetable cooking spray.

Peel and slice potato. Place in a small saucepan with enough water to cover. Bring to a boil, then reduce heat, cover, and cook until tender. Drain, reserving ¾ cup of the potato water.

Mash potato, then add ½ cup mashed potato and honey to reserved potato water, stirring well.

Preheat oven to 375°F.

Sift together flours, baking soda, cream of tartar, and salt into a medium bowl. Stir in oats and currants.

Make a well in the center of the dry ingredients and pour in the potato mixture. Stir until a stiff dough forms. Turn out onto a floured board and knead 1 minute with floured hands. Shape into a ball and place in prepared pan and flatten slightly. With a sharp knife, make a cross slash in the top of the loaf.

Bake for 25 to 35 minutes, or until loaf sounds hollow when tapped.

Serve plain or with fruit butter, jam, honey, or a slice of cheese. Or serve with a hearty soup or stew. For best slicing, cool completely before serving.

Makes 12 servings (Each slice has 2.4 grams total dietary fiber, 116 calories, and 0.6 grams fat.)

though used in some fiber supplements and in low-calorie bread, it does not appear to have any of fiber's beneficial effects.

And you should be sure to increase your fluid intake to the equivalent of six to eight glasses a day. Otherwise, since insoluble fiber acts like a sponge in the intestinal tract, you risk dehydration.

STARCH: THE "FIBER" OF THE FUTURE?

Fiber researchers were puzzled. If low-fiber diets meant a higher incidence of bowel cancer, why did the Japanese get so little bowel cancer? After all, their diet is very low in fiber. An answer emerged: starch. The Japanese may not eat much fiber, but they eat *lots* of starch-rich rice.

Scientists used to think that only dietary fiber escaped digestion in the small intestine. Recently, more accurate measuring techniques have disclosed that a certain amount of starch, aptly named resistant starch, escapes as well. And if starch resists digestion as fiber does, researchers have hypothesized, maybe it has a positive effect on bowel cancer—just as fiber is suspected of doing.

So research is turning toward starch as a possible anticancer substance in the diet. "There is now increasing evidence that starch may be equally important in this whole context," says John Cummings, M.D., a British fiber expert and leading proponent of the starch hypothesis. "You can't explain the distribution of bowel cancer or breast cancer worldwide on the basis of fiber alone. If you put starch into the equation, you can start to do it much better."

Good food sources of starch include potatoes, rice, and whole grains.

Diet Profiles:
Little Changes, Big Benefits

Ever wonder what a nutritionist would say about your diet—but were afraid to ask? Well, here are profiles of five brave souls of widely varying ages and lifestyles who did ask—and they're glad they did.

They discovered what was right and not-so-right about their eating habits. And they learned the Grand Lesson of Practical Nutrition: It usually takes just a little fine-tuning to improve your diet in big ways—ways that are compatible with your lifestyle and your tastes.

The five volunteers wrote down everything they ate for three consecutive days. (They all were concerned about what they ate. But they were hardly nutritional saints—along with salads and skinned chicken, they were occasionally downing beers and candy bars.) Then nutritionists Joan Connors, R.D., and Elaine Blethen, R.D., of the Tufts Nutrient Data Center at the Tufts University School of Medicine in Boston, evaluated the diaries (with the help of a massive computer database) and made recommendations for better health. So here are five profiles in courage . . . with the experts' analyses and tips for revamped nutrition.

Martha, 66, Bookkeeper

"She's done a great job lowering her cholesterol, but she's taken the joy and variety out of eating."

Nutritional Profile • Martha recalls the time when she loved eggs and ate two each day. But about a year ago, her doctor told her that her blood cholesterol was high, hovering around 260. So following her doctor's guidelines, she started stripping cholesterol and saturated fats (which raise cholesterol levels) from her diet. Exit all eggs, red meat, butter, and cheese. She even stopped eating processed crackers and soups that contain saturated vegetable oils, such as coconut oil and palm oil.

Her menu emphasizes poultry, occasional cooked vegetables, and flavored gelatins for dessert.

Assessment • On the plus side, the Tufts nutritionists complimented Martha for significantly reducing her intake of fats. Her daily cholesterol intake for the three days averaged 130 milligrams (200 milligrams is considered a severe restriction). The percentage of calories derived from fat was also ultra-low: 20 percent. (Authorities recommend under 30 percent.)

But there were several points in the minus column. Because she avoids milk and cheese, her intake of calcium averaged 392 milligrams for three days, far below the recommended intake of 800 milligrams (even further below the 1,500 milligrams daily intake some scientists recommend for older women to keep bones strong).

Also, she doesn't eat many fresh fruits or vegetables, so her vitamin A intake is inadequate. And because Martha wants to lose weight, her calorie intake is low—too low, averaging about 1,200 calories per day. But her lifestyle is very sedentary, so her extra pounds won't come off.

Recommendations • "Relax and eat a little more!" advises Joan Connors. "The amount of fat in a cracker is so insignificant that it's not worth giving up."

Martha needs to expand her protein repertoire. She's relying too much on poultry, especially processed poultry, which she sometimes eats twice daily. She should include in her diet fish, lean beef, pork, and low-fat dairy products.

She needs to eat more fresh fruits and vegetables instead of flavored gelatins, which have little nutritional value.

She should seek out more calcium-rich foods, such as low-fat dairy products, and breads and puddings made with milk. If she can't get two to three servings of calcium-rich foods each day, she should consider a calcium supplement.

She needs to consider rechanneling energy into exercise, instead of severe dietary restrictions. When she exercises, she'll be able to eat more and still lower her blood cholesterol.

Andre, 38, Contractor/Carpenter

"He burns a lot of calories on the job, and that may be his excuse to eat more than he needs. But he needs to pay more attention to low-fat eating, to maintain a healthy heart."

Nutritional Profile • "I want to eat healthfully, and I'm aware of it when I don't," says Andre. "But I need to have my little sins, in moderation."

Much of Andre's diet is not only not sinful, it's healthy and appealing as well. He brown-bags a thoughtful workman's lunch with a tuna salad, turkey, or other protein-filled sandwich, fruits, fresh juice, and yogurt or potato chips on the side or as afternoon snacks. For dinner, he often concocts marvelous, albeit enormous, meals for himself and his lucky wife. Andre's "little sins" include occasional chocolate cookies, ice cream, and a daily cola.

Assessment • On the plus side, the nutritionists complimented Andre for eating a wide variety of quality foods. His intake of most nutrients is above recommended levels, except sometimes for calcium.

Another plus: Andre's snacks are usually good foods, though occasionally there are soft drinks or sweets.

In the minus column is the fact that Andre's calorie intake averaged 3,339. "Because he works physically, it could be okay, but it's probably a little high," says Connors. "The average male needs about 2,700 calories a day."

The Tufts nutritionists also spotted one big miscue—he eats two croissants for breakfast. Those two pastries pack more of the bad things than he thought—about 55 grams of fat, 1,400 milligrams of sodium, 205 milligrams of cholesterol and 857 calories in all! That's more fat, sodium, and calories than in one of Andre's hearty weekend breakfasts, which include three slices of bacon and two fried eggs!

Also negative was his percentage of calories from fat—a high 46 percent. And his cholesterol intake was the highest of any of the volunteers, an average of 828 milligrams daily.

Recommendations • He should aim to cut 50 to 100 calories per day simply by controlling his portion size—and preparing less enormous meals.

Reducing fat is a priority for Andre. Reducing fat intake to 30 percent of calories will be a significant task, but cutting out the croissants would make a huge dent. Instead of two croissants, he could have two bagels or four pieces of toast with jelly, peanut butter, low-fat cottage cheese, or yogurt, or cereal with low-fat milk. He should moderate his red meat intake, too.

Helen, 58, Schoolteacher

"Helen has demonstrated that it's possible to eat out frequently and still have a healthy diet."

Nutritional Profile • Helen works harder than many women half her age. She wakes up at 6:00 A.M. and heads for a diner for her standard breakfast of two eggs with toast. She's at her desk, as a teacher in a large public high school, by 8:00. Helen packs fruits, vegetables, and yogurt for lunch, or sometimes orders soup and salad from the school cafeteria. After school she takes an hour to exercise at a health spa. She almost always eats dinner with her husband at a Chinese, Italian, or Middle Eastern restaurant.

Helen considers breakfast the most important meal of her day. "It gives me the energy that I need," she says. "And I also believe that a good breakfast really helps me stay thin because I never have to snack later." At dinner, she chooses carefully. "Under no circumstances do I order fried foods." Instead, she asks for fish or chicken and pasta dishes. She finishes her dinners with decaffeinated coffee.

Assessment • Helen got a big plus rating from the nutritionists because her "food choices are wonderful," says Joan Connors. "Usually, people who eat out frequently eat more calories and more fat." Over three days, her daily calorie intake averaged a sensible 1,600. Her fat intake averaged just under 30 percent of calories.

She also got good marks because she eats fresh fruits and vegetables twice a day or more. Helen brings them along in her lunch, orders a green salad with dinner, or gets her vegetables in a Chinese stir-fry. This keeps her vitamin A and C levels high.

Helen's diet does have one major flaw: the two breakfast eggs. They helped bring her cholesterol intake to a daily average of 724 milligrams, more than twice recommended levels.

And another potential problem: If she weren't taking a supplement, she wouldn't meet the daily requirement for calcium, since her average calcium intake from food was only 516 milligrams With the supplement, her intake was 1,182 milligrams, still short of the 1,500 milligrams some experts recommend for postmenopausal women.

Recommendations • Nutritionist Elaine Blethen recommends that Helen order one egg instead of two, twice a week only. (She could eat another slice of toast to make up for the second egg.)

She should eat more calcium-rich foods. All she needs is two more dairy servings each day. If she forgoes the calcium foods, she should definitely continue taking her calcium supplement.

Martin, 49, Advertising Executive

"You can see from his record that his work controls how he eats. He needs to reach a balance."

Nutritional Profile • It's true, Martin says: "My work rules my life. I know about good foods, but my work is a higher priority than eating correctly."

The conflict shows in Martin's three-day food record. A typical morning starts with a 6:30 A.M. cafe-au-lait (half coffee and half whole milk). "I haven't eaten breakfast in 20 years. It makes me feel stuffed and sleepy," he says. But later in the morning, if he's in a business meeting where pastries are served, he'll down one or two.

Usually his first meal of the day isn't until noon or early afternoon. Lunch is where Martin's health-consciousness shows. He helps himself to a healthy salad, with a few ounces of cheese or meat.

Martin feels his biggest nutritional problem is midnight snacking. "I often wind up doing creative work late at night. Spinning out strategies, I become very hungry, and my food choices are very poor: beer, wine, ice cream."

Assessment • Martin got a plus because he eats salads daily, making his intake of vitamin A very high.

However, he scored on the negative side because coffee with nothing else is a poor way to start the day—caffeine can irritate the stomach, maybe set the stage for an ulcer. Skipping breakfast can also reduce productivity and probably contributes to Martin's uncontrollable late-night munchies.

He also got minuses because he drinks whole milk and eats pastries, ice cream, and red meat frequently, thus his percentage of calories from fat was high: 39 percent. And despite the fatty foods, his total calories are low—averaging 1,950 calories, compared to a recommended average of around 2,700.

Recommendations • Martin needs to cut back on fats and add more calories from complex carbohydrates. Calories from complex carbohydrates are less likely to be turned into body fat than calories from fatty foods.

He might try more breads. Martin's food record reveals that he avoids breads, which he thinks of as high-calorie foods. But he can afford the calories, and he needs the iron and B vitamins grains offer.

He should give breakfast a chance. If he's really not hungry first thing, he could aim for a midmorning snack of toast or fruit. He could also bring fruit to business meetings to help him resist high-fat pastries.

At home, he could stock up on good snacks to make it easier to resist poor late-night food choices. Some healthier snack foods: popcorn, crackers with low-fat cheese, fruit, low-fat yogurt, and juices.

Karen, 24, Law Student

"Karen engages in a popular eating style, called grazing. It satisfies her appetite and helps her keep her weight under control. Unfortunately, she's sacrificing good nutrition."

Nutritional Profile • Karen is concerned about eating right and maintaining her weight. But she also has a grueling class and study schedule and feels that she doesn't have much time to prepare meals. Result: Her eating runs to extremes, between good and not-so-good foods.

She often doesn't eat breakfast until midmorning, and it's usually something quick: a pastry or a piece of fruit. Lunch is great: a salad or a turkey or tuna sandwich. Then in the afternoon, the cravings strike. Ice cream and candy are frequent choices. Dinner is dictated by her social and study partners: She often shares in the group's pizza or fried chicken, taking only small portions.

Assessment • On the plus side, the nutritionists felt that one thing that Karen is doing right is eating plenty of salads. They bolster her intake of vitamins A and C and fiber.

In the minus column, Karen's total calorie intake is low, even with her sweet and fatty snacks. The three-day average was only 1,399 calories daily, well below the 1,800 recommended for active young women. She takes meager portions of nutrient-rich foods like proteins, grains, and fruits.

Also, a high percentage of Karen's calories comes from fat—her daily average was 46 percent. And her iron intake is low because she eats so little meat. She doesn't eat many dairy products either, and her calcium intake doesn't meet the 800-milligram requirement.

Also a minus was the fact that Karen drinks several diet soft drinks each day, including one in the morning. Colas are usually irritating to an empty stomach. They're also a diuretic, ultimately reducing fluids in the body. And soft drinks contain phosphorus: Too much can upset the body's balance of calcium and phosphorus, important in building and maintaining strong bone.

Recommendations • Karen needs to focus on eating fewer fats, but more calories overall. She can get the extra calories from grains and protein. (They'll also improve her iron levels.)

She should avoid breakfast pastries—they contain too much fat. And she needs to choose nutrient-rich, low-fat snacks, such as fruits, yogurt, raisins, or popcorn.

She should cut back on soda and drink water or juice instead.

Karen needs to eat more calcium- and vitamin-rich foods. A supplement would help her.

Mind Your Monos, Help Your Heart

Right out of left field has come a scientific discovery that may change forever our ideas about a heart-healthy diet. To everyone's surprise, new research has suggested that (of all things) a fat that has been ignored and underrated may be an ally in the war on heart disease.

The new heart-friendly factor is something called mono-unsaturated fat. It's always been part of our diets (It's abundant in olive oil, avocados, and nuts). But now scientists are learning that in the right amounts "monos" may do our arteries a lot of good. So what do researchers know so far about monos? And how should we incorporate these fats into a healthy-heart diet designed to keep fats low? Here are the answers.

The Mediterranean Secret

The first clue about the mono/heart connection came from a peculiar fact: Among people who live around the Mediterranean, heart disease is, by most standards, uncommon. Mediterraneans die from heart disease only half as often as Americans do. Yet, as Americans do, Greeks and Italians get about 40 percent of their calories from fat, the arch-enemy of arteries.

Why the difference? Since heart attacks can have multiple causes, many factors could account for it, but certain scientists suspected the key difference was dietary.

Scott M. Grundy, M.D., Ph.D., director of the Center for Human Nutrition at the University of Texas Southwestern Medical Center and a leading cholesterol researcher, set out to investigate the effects of various levels and kinds of fat in the diet. In 1985 he and a colleague, Fred H. Mattson, Ph.D., retired professor at the University of California in San Diego, produced evidence that sent members of the scientific and medical worlds back to their labs to reexamine facts about fats' effects on cholesterol that up until then had seemed well established. Their study provided evidence that monounsaturated fats lowered cholesterol. This was ground-breaking news, since until then most scientists believed only polyunsaturated fats had a cholesterol-lowering effect.

In a 1986 study, Dr. Grundy examined the effects of monos further. He fed 11 patients three liquid diets that varied in fat content. For four weeks, his patients drank a liquid that looked and tasted much like a vanilla milk shake. Like a real milk shake, it was high in saturated fat. For another four weeks, the patients drank a similar shake, only this time it was low in fat and high in carbohydrates. During yet another four-week period, they drank a third shake, high in monounsaturated fat.

The patients' blood cholesterol level peaked on the saturated-fat diet. That was no surprise. Doctors agree that certain types of saturated fat (found mostly in rich dairy products, meat fat, and coconut oil) raise blood cholesterol substantially.

In contrast, the low-fat, high-carbohydrate diet significantly lowered total cholesterol. Again, no surprise. Cutting fat (especially saturated fat) and adding carbohydrates (especially fruits, vegetables, and grains) have long been the standard prescriptions for lowering cholesterol. Dr. Grundy also found that this low-fat, high-carb diet lowered both major types of cholesterol: LDL (low-density lipoprotein), the "bad" cholesterol that jams arteries, and HDL (high-density lipoprotein), the "good" cholesterol that helps clear arteries.

As for the monounsaturated-fat diet, it also lowered total cholesterol—but even more than the low-fat diet!

Even more earth-shattering was how the monounsaturated fats lowered cholesterol: They selectively lowered the bad cholesterol, leaving the good kind intact (*New England Journal of Medicine*).

Since Dr. Grundy conducted his study, three tests have independently confirmed that monounsaturated fats lower LDL and leave HDL unscathed. "Diets high in monounsaturated fatty acids appear to be as protective against [heart disease] as those low in total fat," Dr. Grundy concluded in the journal *Circulation*.

How do these findings explain why Greeks and Italians have such healthy hearts? The connection is that mainstay of Mediterranean cuisine—olive oil. Olive oil is about 75 percent monounsaturated fats.

A study published by Italian doctors offers some of the most concrete evidence of olive oil's impact. The doctors fed 11 young volunteers two diets—this time consisting of real food instead of laboratory "milk shakes." One diet was enriched with olive oil served Italian style: with salad, boiled vegetables, bread, and pasta. The other was a standard low-fat diet. In this study, the olive oil diet lowered LDL even more than the low-fat diet, without changing HDL (*American Journal of Clinical Nutrition*).

Perspective on Monos

The news about olive oil and monounsaturated fats is exciting, though there are still some unanswered questions. Because the studies are small, some researchers wonder if the results really apply to everyone—or if just some people benefit from higher mono intake. Others ask whether monos actually decrease LDL or whether LDL lowering is the result of replacing saturated fats with unsaturated ones. They warn that while replacing saturated fat with small quantities of olive oil cuts LDL, olive oil is, after all, pure fat. In excess, any fat promotes obesity, and obesity is associated with increased LDL.

Of course, monos in the form of olive oil have been a staple for centuries with no known harmful effects.

ALL ABOUT OLIVE OIL

Olive oils differ in flavor, bouquet, and color, just as wines do. Some people save top-of-the-line oil for salads, when the oil's flavor is least adorned by other flavors, and use lesser grades of oil in more highly seasoned cooking.

Virgin designates the top grade of olive oil. By international agreement, it may not be mixed with refined oils and still be considered virgin. Within this designation are three categories: *Extra-virgin* olive oil has "absolutely perfect flavor," according to the International Olive and Olive Oil Agreement of 1986. And extra-virgin oil must have no more than 1 percent free oleic acid. *Fine virgin* oil meets the same standards, except it may have up to 1.5 percent free oleic acid. *Semi-fine* or ordinary virgin oil (labels say simply "virgin") must have "good" flavor and no more than 3 percent free oleic acid.

Three other designations are worth knowing. *Refined* oil comes from the processing of oil that's too high in acidity or has an "off" flavor. Refining the oil removes extra acid—along with color, odor, and much of the flavor. *Pure* olive oil is a mixture of refined and virgin oils. Manufacturers add enough virgin oil to give the mixture the desired flavor and aroma. It doesn't necessarily taste weaker than extra virgin oil. "Some pure olive oil seems to have a very 'olive-y' taste," says Richard Sullivan, executive vice president of the Olive Oil Group, an association of importers and marketers. "Extra virgins sometimes have a more delicate flavor. It's like the difference between a fine wine and a table wine."

Light, the newest variety, is named not for its caloric content but for its flavor. Light is pure olive oil made with very little virgin oil. It's aimed at consumers who want to use olive oil with only a hint of the olive taste.

Making the Most of Monos

Considering the evidence, what should we do about this monounsaturated breakthrough?

For weight maintenance and all-around good health, most people should benefit from eating a low-fat diet—one that contains less than 30 percent of calories from fat. That diet is easy to maintain by focusing on fresh fruits and vegetables, whole grains, lean meat, skinless poultry, and fish, avoiding butter, and choosing low-fat and nonfat dairy products.

Once you've trimmed your diet to these essentials, "supplement" with about 2 to 3 tablespoons of olive oil a day—or an equivalent amount of mono-rich foods (see "Mind Your Monos"). That doesn't mean dumping on the oil. Rather, use monos to replace some of the other fats remaining in your diet.

Try using flavorful olive oil on salads and pasta. If you're cooking something that doesn't go with olive oil, try canola oil (a new unflavored mono oil made from rapeseed). Other polyunsaturated fats—corn, safflower, sunflower-seed, and soybean oils, for example—are important, too, and should be used whenever they can substitute for butter or lard. Polyunsaturated oils contain linoleic acid, an essential fatty acid our bodies can't make. A tablespoon of polyunsaturated vegetable oil per day supplies just the right amount of linoleic acid.

MIND YOUR MONOS

A tablespoon of olive oil averages almost 10 grams of monounsaturated fat. You can also get the same amount from the following nutritious alternatives.

- $3\frac{1}{2}$ tablespoons almonds
- $1\frac{1}{2}$ tablespoons almond butter
- $\frac{1}{2}$ avocado
- 4 teaspoons canola oil
- 3 tablespoons hazelnuts
- 2 tablespoons macadamia nuts
- $\frac{1}{4}$ cup peanuts
- $2\frac{1}{2}$ tablespoons peanut butter
- $1\frac{1}{2}$ tablespoons peanut oil
- $3\frac{1}{2}$ tablespoons pecans
- $\frac{1}{4}$ cup pistachios

Protein:
Cut Down on Beefing Up

By George L. Blackburn, M.D., Ph.D.

Until recent years, the place of honor on nearly every American dinner plate was reserved for a large piece of meat. Whether it was a juicy steak or burger, a turkey drumstick or a rack of ribs, no supper seemed complete without the meat dominating, with smaller portions of other foods—rice, potatoes, cooked vegetables, or salad—surrounding it like admirers.

How did nutritionists justify this way of eating? Protein!

Protein was considered the most important nutrient, and not entirely without reason. After all, protein is in every cell of the body; protein builds and rebuilds everything from muscles and bones to blood vessels, hormones, hair, and fingernails.

Scientists believed that the best sources of protein were the animal sources—meat, fowl, fish, and eggs. This, too, seemed like a logical conclusion. Protein is composed of 22 nitrogen-containing compounds called amino acids. Any given vegetable product contains some—but not all—of the amino acids. Most meats, on the other hand, contain all the amino acids, including the nine essential ones that our body can't produce itself and must get from foods.

Shattering the Myths

Unfortunately, some of the conclusions drawn from these facts have turned out to be wrong. We now have a better understanding of how our body derives and uses protein. Let's debunk those old myths.

Myth #1: Americans Need More Protein • The fact is, most Americans eat too much protein. The amount required for health is only 6 to 8 percent of our daily calories. Nowadays, the American average is closer to 15 percent of calories from protein, which is probably fine as an upper limit. Many people, of course, are eating much more.

41

What are the consequences of consuming too much protein? A general problem is that high-protein foods are often rich in calories. And animal proteins, especially, are likely to be high in calories and fats.

Excessive protein also takes a toll on the kidneys. The kidneys excrete protein breakdown products. If you give your kidneys more protein than they can handle—particularly animal protein, which is more difficult to process—it wears them down. Americans' obsession with getting enough protein may explain the fact that renal (kidney) disease is so common here.

Myth #2: Meat, Eggs, and Dairy Products Are the Best Sources • Many scientists used to believe that "animal-grade" protein was superior to "vegetable grade." Now we know that a mixture of animal and vegetable proteins is used most efficiently by the body.

For example, eggs were once thought to be the perfect protein source, because they contain all the amino acids. But scientists have found that if you replace a third of the egg protein with potato protein, the body actually uses it more efficiently for fuel or to build tissue.

Efficient utilization isn't the only argument in favor of deriving a greater share of your protein from vegetable sources. There are the health concerns about animal proteins. As we've mentioned, meats often contain too much fat and too many calories. Research also shows that a diet high in animal protein may interfere with the absorption of certain minerals—particularly calcium—from the bowel, and may cause excretion of more minerals in the urine.

Myth #3: Protein Builds Muscle, Not Fat • The body does use protein to build muscle. But if you get 6 percent of your calories from protein, that meets your muscle-building needs. And, the fact is, any extra protein not burned for fuel will become the same thing an extra piece of cake becomes: *fat*.

The way to build muscle is not to beef up your protein intake; it's to pump iron. You may need to consume 100 to 200 extra calories each day to build and sustain the extra tissue—

but you'll want to distribute those calories among complex carbohydrates, proteins, and fat.

Myth #4: Vegetable Sources Must Be Balanced at Each Meal to Create a Complete Protein ● The fact is, it's not necessary to mix vegetable sources at the same meal to get a balance of amino acids. We now know that eating a variety of vegetables, grains, and beans on the same day allows the body to create complete proteins because we have internal reserves of amino acids.

Most vegetarians who eat a wide range of food have almost no problem meeting their protein requirements. However, there are some vegetarians who should be concerned about getting adequate protein: pregnant and nursing women. Also, if children are being raised on a vegetarian regimen, a pediatrician should be consulted.

The Bottom Line

What should a sensible, moderate-protein diet look like? Any well-balanced diet should derive most of its calories— about 50 to 60 percent—from complex carbohydrates, and no more than 30 percent of calories from fat.

That leaves about 15 percent of calories from protein. And of that 15 percent, no more than half should come from animal sources.

Here's an easy rule of thumb to follow: Women should limit daily servings of meat, fowl, or fish to no more than two servings, 3 to 4 ounces in weight (about one loin lamb chop, or one-half chicken breast, or four steamed jumbo shrimp). Men can afford a little more protein: two 4- to 6-ounce servings per day.

The best way to translate those numbers into practice is to rethink your plate. Stop making the meat, fowl, or fish the center of attention at lunches and dinners. Instead, think of meats as condiments, to add flavor to a stir-fry, spaghetti sauce, or casserole, for example. Vegetables and grains should dominate your plate. When you do serve a piece of meat, train yourself and your family to be pleased with smaller portions.

If you have a special concern, such as kidney problems, talk to your physician or a registered dietitian. She or he can help you analyze your diet for protein content, and suggest ways to improve it.

Top Food Picks from the Nutrition Pros

Science has gleaned a lot of useful information from studying the average American's diet. But there's also something to be learned from the diet of not-so-average Americans: specifically, people highly schooled in the field of nutrition—people on the forefront of food and nutrition science.

Here, five leading researchers reveal the "inside information" that has affected their own diets. They tell which research, specifically, has changed how they eat and why. Do they follow any fundamental principles? Do they use any "tricks of the trade" in structuring their own diets? In most cases, the answer is yes.

Sheldon Reiser, Ph.D., is research leader of the Carbohydrate Nutrition Laboratory of the USDA Beltsville Human Nutrition Research Center. His group investigates the metabolic effects of dietary carbohydrates—such as starches, sugars, and fiber—and how they affect risk factors associated with diseases such as diabetes, heart disease, and cancer.

"What I have learned from my research primarily is that genetics controls most of how a food component produces a metabolic effect in our bodies. I would say that environmental factors, such as diet, contribute only 25 to 30 percent to your ultimate disease susceptibility. But I feel that anything I can do to prevent disease, including making changes in this 25 to 30 percent, is to my benefit.

"So I've made it a point to know my 'metabolic profile'— my body's nutritional status as reflected in certain factors in my blood. I'm lucky enough to be able to check that at work, but most people can find out their profile by having their doctor do a blood test. The type of blood lipids, or fats, you have will give you an idea of what foods you should be concerned about. If your triglycerides are high, for example, that means you're getting too much sugar and alcohol. If your cholesterol levels are high, you have to look at the saturated fat and cholesterol in your diet.

"From my metabolic profile, I can see that I would be more sensitive to the effect of saturated fat and cholesterol than sugar. So I'm very careful about my fat intake. The main source of protein in my diet is usually poultry or fish. I also rely on low-fat cottage cheese and polyunsaturated cooking oils.

"I do eat sweets, though, and I find ice milk is a good choice for me—it has the sweetness I want, but the fat is reduced compared to ice cream.

"I'm also very aware of the fact that cruciferous vegetables are good for you. Of all of the anticancer foods, they seem to be the ones that are thought of most highly as possible preventives of bowel cancer. When I look at the list of cancers that could get me, that one is pretty high up. (Since I don't smoke, I'm not too concerned about lung cancer.) I think the information on cruciferous vegetables is pretty solid. And I just happen to like brussels sprouts and cabbage. [Other members of the crucifer family include broccoli, kale, kohlrabi, rutabagas and turnips.] They're low in calories, high in fiber, and a fairly good source of vitamins, too.

"Overall, I'm trying to create the best environment I can to live life in the most enjoyable way I can."

Ritva Butrum, Ph.D., is chief of the Diet and Cancer Branch, Division of Cancer Prevention and Control, of the National Cancer Institute. The branch supports research on dietary fiber, vitamin A, carotenoids, and other dietary components. It has also funded the "Women's Health Trial," a multicenter, clinical intervention trial that investigated the effect of a low-fat diet in women at increased risk of breast cancer.

"My work with cancer prevention during the last five years has really made an impact on me. Before that I really didn't think about prevention.

"We promote lowering fat intake and increasing fiber intake to help prevent cancer, and I practice what I preach. But reducing the risk of cancer isn't the only reason I've changed my diet. A low-fat diet lowers the risk of heart disease as well. And there's heart disease in my family. So I'm hoping that my diet will be protective overall.

"I follow our own guidelines to reduce the fat in my diet: using low-fat milk products, buying leaner cuts of meat and trimming the fat, using cooking methods that don't add fat, such as broiling, stewing and baking, and using less oil—I use only half the salad dressing I used to.

"To make sure I'm getting plenty of fiber in my diet, I eat only whole grain bread, and I've increased my intake of cereal, fruit, and vegetables. One thing that helps is not eating meat at lunch. Instead, I'll plan something like yogurt and fruit with cereal mixed in.

"I've also added more carbohydrates to my diet. If you cut down your fat, you have to replace those calories with something. So I eat more potatoes, pasta, and whole grain bread.

"I'm convinced that people should go with these dietary changes. The research is very strong. As for myself, I'm happy about the bonus I get for modifying my diet: I simply feel better."

Michael F. Holick, M.D., Ph.D., is director of the Vitamin D, Skin and Bone Research Laboratory at Boston University School of Medicine. His research is increasing our understanding of how the sun produces vitamin D in the skin, and how vitamin D nutrition and bone disease are interrelated in the elderly. In order to develop a treatment for psoriasis, he is also studying how vitamin D interacts with skin cells.

"There are several principles that I use to structure my own diet and that of my family. From all the scientific literature I've read, it seems that for certain individuals there is a clear association between salt intake and hypertension. So we have a no-added-salt diet. We don't exclude foods that contain salt, but we don't add salt to our food.

"There is also a very clear association between the amount of saturated fat in your diet and heart disease. For that reason, we've made the decision to decrease our saturated-fat intake. I have a three-year-old daughter and a nine-year-old son. If there's a family history of heart disease, even children can start laying down cholesterol in their blood vessels—and there is heart disease in my family. So most of the week we eat chicken without the skin, or fish. And when we do eat red meat, it's lean.

"I think the data on fish oil look encouraging. It appears to me that a high-fish diet may be one of the reasons that Eskimos have a low incidence of cardiovascular disease. The research hasn't affected my diet, however. I already follow a low-fat diet, and I know that my cholesterol level isn't high, so I don't think I need to eat any more fish.

"We are concerned about calcium intake, though, especially for my wife and our growing children. So each of us usually drinks somewhere between three and four glasses of 1 percent milk a day.

"We've also increased our fiber intake. There is pretty good evidence that increasing the amount of fiber in the diet decreases the risk of diverticulosis. Fiber may also play a role in decreasing the incidence of colon cancer—there's enough data to suggest that increasing your intake is certainly not unreasonable. So our cereal in the morning is high fiber. And we routinely have large salads for dinner and fruit throughout the day.

"I love to garden. So from April through November, our plates are filled with lots of very nice vegetables that are organically grown. We're getting a lot of vitamins and minerals and fiber just by virtue of eating what we grow.

"My own research with vitamin D hasn't really affected my diet. I get enough sunlight from my exposure out in the garden. And it's my feeling based on our work that it is casual exposure to sunlight that provides our vitamin D requirement for the most part, and that healthy young adults and children store enough to get through the winter."

George A. Bray, M.D., is professor of medicine at the University of Southern California. His research into why animals get fat is helping us to understand causes of human obesity.

"The only thing I really make an effort to do through diet is keep my weight stable, because the evidence suggests that being overweight is hazardous to your health. Obesity has been linked to heart disease, high blood pressure, diabetes, and gallbladder disease.

"So I weigh myself regularly. If I find I've gained a couple of pounds, I eat less but remain active. My action relates to the entire stream of research that suggests that you get fat largely by taking in more energy than you expend.

"I find that the easiest approach is to eliminate the snack foods that I tend to eat in large amounts, such as crackers and cheese, salted peanuts, and ice cream. My weight is now exactly where it was more than 35 years ago."

Walter Mertz, M.D., is director of the USDA Beltsville Human Nutrition Research Center. As a trace-element researcher, he was co-discoverer of the essential role of chromium. His work now spans many areas of nutrition.

"If I had to summarize everything that I know in nutrition, it would come to this: balance. Whenever you single out any particular component of your diet to the exclusion of others, you get away from that.

"So my wife and I practice this kind of moderation by striving to eat a wide variety of foods. We try to eat different vegetables and fruits every day, rather than just the same ones over and over, for example. By eating a varied diet, you don't get too little of anything, but you also don't get too much of anything undesirable, such as fat.

"One thing that helps get variety into our diet is that we are a little bit nuts about fresh things. We love to eat fruits and vegetables as they come into season. One of the things we really enjoy, for example, is the first fresh strawberries. Or the first fresh pears, or whatever. Of course, during winter we also eat things that are not necessarily in season here. We'll eat fresh fruit and vegetables at just about every meal.

"I have never taken any trace-mineral supplements. Everything that I have learned about trace minerals reinforces my belief that it's the variety in your food choices that gives you the best guarantee that you get your requirements of those and all the other important nutrients. The only time we take a daily vitamin supplement is when we're on a long trip and don't have control over our diet.

"Here is another principle of good nutrition, which is entirely my own: We shouldn't alter our diets out of scientific conviction alone—but also because we enjoy eating the new way. I firmly and deeply believe that enjoyment of food is a very important part of eating and diet."

The Newest News on Omega-3's

By George L. Blackburn, M.D., Ph.D.

You've seen plenty of headlines about fish oil in recent years. Perhaps you've wondered: Is this a short-lived fad? Or is it a significant nutritional discovery?

My bet is that, as time goes on, you'll be hearing even more about fish oil. Scientists are nearing a consensus on its benefits. I predict that, in a year or two, the government and professional nutrition associations will even issue guidelines for recommended minimum (and maximum) fish-oil intake.

Why? Fish oils belong to a category of unsaturated fats called the omega-3's. My review of the evidence leads me to believe that increasing the proportion of omega-3's in the diet may influence the course of arthritis, heart disease, and even cancer.

The whole question of what kind of fat you should eat, and how much, can be confusing. Nutritionists agree that most Americans need to cut back their total fat intake—regardless of what kind of fat it is—to fewer than 30 percent calories from fat.

Good Fat, Bad Fat?

Once you've lowered the overall fat level, it's time to start thinking about the type of fat you're eating. Since the 1970s, Americans have begun to think in terms of "good" and "bad" fats. The bad fats, of course, are the saturated fats—the kinds of fat in animal products. Saturated fats raise blood cholesterol levels and promote heart disease. The "better" fats are the unsaturated fats, including most fats from vegetable sources. (Of course, any fat is bad if you eat too much of it.)

Polyunsaturates Aren't Created Equal

Now scientists are learning that the polyunsaturates do not all have the same effect in the body. Polyunsaturates that come from vegetable sources are called the omega-6's. Another kind of polyunsaturated fats, the omega-3's, come primarily from deep-water fish, although they're also found in small quantities in a few plants.

Today Americans eat a diet that is unprecedentedly low in omega-3's. Before World War II, most livestock wandered free, eating wild grasses that contained significant amounts of omega-3's. When we ate their meat, we consumed omega-3's. So the ratio of omega-6 to omega-3 fats in the American diet was probably about 3 to 1 or 2 to 1.

But now livestock eat grain-based feed, which contains little or no omega-3. Our main source of omega-3 has been shut off. If we don't eat much fish—and many Americans don't—then we get very little omega-3. The ratio of omega-6 to omega-3 in our diet has increased to about 20 to 1.

My hypothesis is that this imbalance has left our blood more prone to inflammation—more "activated." Omega-3's act differently from omega-6's on the cellular, biochemical level. This difference may account for the epidemic of diseases, such as heart disease, cancer, and arthritis. Restoring a more balanced ratio of omega-6 to omega-3 may make a difference in preventing, and, to some degree, treating those diseases and other ailments.

Omega-3 and the Heart

Research into the diet of Greenland Eskimos first triggered interest in omega-3's and cardiac health. In the mid-1970s, researchers discovered that the Eskimos have less heart disease than Western populations, even though their diet is higher in fat. The difference: The Greenlanders' dietary fat comes from the meat of walrus, seal, whale, and oily cold-water fish, which are rich in omega-3's.

Since then, animal and human studies have suggested a variety of mechanisms by which omega-3's may benefit the heart, compared to omega-6's.

Consumption of omega-6 fats leads to production in the blood cells of a substance called thromboxane, which makes blood cells stiffer and more susceptible to getting stuck in narrow arteries, helping to build up the plaque that can ultimately be deadly.

By contrast, omega-3 fatty acids inhibit the formation of thromboxane and encourage production of another substance, prostacyclin, which opens the pathways. Less clotting means a reduced likelihood of atherosclerosis or, ultimately, heart attack.

Several studies have demonstrated significant benefits for heart patients when they increased their intake of omega-3's. One of the most important recent studies was conducted at the Dallas Veterans Administration Hospital, and reported in the *New England Journal of Medicine.*

The Dallas researchers were curious about the effects of fish oil on men scheduled to undergo an angioplasty procedure, in which plaque-clogged arteries are opened by passing a tube through them. One problem with angioplasty is that, in the months after the procedure, the vessels can accumulate more plaque and close up again, a process called restenosis.

The researchers took a group of 82 men who were scheduled for angioplasty. Half the men were given the conventional therapy, which included aspirin and an anticlotting drug. The other half received the aspirin and drug, plus 18 fish-oil capsules (3.2 grams) daily. The treatment began seven days before angioplasty and continued for six months after.

After three to four months, the researchers found that restenosis of the blood vessels occurred in 36 percent of men in the control group, but in only 16 percent of the men who received the fish-oil supplementation.

Other studies suggest that fish oil may help prevent and treat a variety of coronary problems, including hypertension, angina, atherosclerosis, and heart attack.

The Cancer Connection

There are three important stages of cancer development and growth. First comes the genetic mutation, in which a regular cell transforms into a cancer cell. After that mutation, the cell can just lie there for an indefinite period—or it can "turn on" and grow. The third step is metastasis, in which the cancer spreads from the primary location.

Most scientists agree that growth and spread can be influenced by calories and fat in the diet. However, scientists do not agree as to which is most important: total calories, total fat, type of calories, or type of fat.

It is my belief that the type of fat makes a difference, and that increasing the ratio of omega-3 to omega-6 can inhibit the growth and spread of cancer. There are about ten different hypotheses as to how this could happen. One possibility is that omega-3's may improve the immune system's recognition of cancer cells, so it can kill cancer cells before they have a chance to grow.

The theory that omega-3's may influence cancer development is based almost entirely on animal studies. Experiments with rats have shown that fish-oil supplementation reduces cancer incidence or shrinks tumors. We don't have the human studies yet to prove whether this is true for us. More research is badly needed in this area.

What to Do

I'm not advocating that you run out and buy crates of fish oil. But there are things you can do to improve the ratio of omega-3 to omega-6 in your diet.

Step one is to eat less total fat. If you're not on a low-fat diet, start now, for your health's sake. That means cutting out fatty meats, whole-milk products, and fat-laden processed foods.

You can get plenty of fish oil into your diet without supplements by eating four to five servings of deep-water fish each week. (Deep-water fish include salmon, mackerel, tuna, halibut, and water-packed sardines.) But if you fry that fish, or buy oil-packed sardines, you're a dead duck! The omega-6 in those products will drown out the omega-3.

Go easy on most vegetable oils. There are, however, some vegetable oils that contain low levels of omega-6's and appreciable amounts of omega-3's: canola oil, made from rapeseed, and linseed oil.

What about fish-oil supplements? Many people ask me this question, but I won't make a general recommendation. I believe that's a task for the National Institutes of Health, the Food and Drug Administration, the American Heart Association, and the American Cancer Society. We should let our doctors, our dietitians, and these agencies and organizations know that we want more information on the ways omega-3's can benefit our health.

Diet Strategies That Heal

50 Top Cancer-Fighting Foods

Eat right, avoid cancer. While that might sound a little simplistic, it may actually be pretty close to the mark.

Top researchers now believe that you can help prevent some kinds of cancer by consistently making the right diet choices. The American Cancer Society, for example, feels the scientific evidence is strong enough to recommend that we eat plenty of cabbage-family (cruciferous) vegetables, vitamin C, vitamin A/beta-carotene, and fiber, and that we minimize our intake of fat, alcohol, and smoked foods. And while the jury's still out, evidence is also casting vitamin E, selenium, and calcium in anticancer roles.

Food Factors against Cancer

How do we know that certain food factors may offer cancer protection? Here's a brief review of the evidence:

Cruciferous, or Cabbage-Family, Vegetables • Some studies of large groups of people (population or epidemiologic studies) have suggested that consumption of these vegetables may reduce the risk of cancer of the gastrointestinal and respiratory tracts. In lab animals, they seem to prevent chemically induced cancer. Cruciferous vegetables include broccoli, brussels sprouts, cabbage, cauliflower, and kale.

Vitamin C • Population studies seem to indicate that people whose diets are rich in citrus fruits and vegetables that contain vitamin C are less likely to get cancer of the stomach and esophagus. (It's not clear, however, whether vitamin C or some other component of the foods exerts the protective effect.) Preliminary studies have shown that vitamin C may combat genetically induced colon polyps. People with polyps are at greater risk for developing colon cancer.

Vitamin A/Beta-Carotene • Many studies have suggested that vitamin A and its relatives, especially beta-carotene, may have anticancer activity. Several population studies indicate that diets high in beta-carotene or vitamin A may lower the risk of cancers of the larynx, esophagus, and lung. Others suggest a protective effect in the stomach, colon, and cervix. And animal studies demonstrate that vitamin A inhibits precancerous changes—and in some cases, cancer—in the prostate, bladder, and breast. While vitamin A is toxic in high doses, beta-carotene, a precursor found in fruits and vegetables, is not.

Fiber • There is a lot of evidence that colon cancer is less common in populations that eat a diet high in fiber.

Low Fat Content • Studies in humans and with laboratory animals suggest that excessive fat intake increases the chance of developing cancers of the breast, colon, and prostate. And a high-fat diet contributes to obesity, which has been linked to cancers of the uterus, gallbladder, breast, and colon. About 40 percent of the calories Americans eat come from fat. Many health agencies recommend reducing that to 30 percent or below.

Vitamin E • A recent study of over 21,000 men linked a high blood level of vitamin E to a reduced overall risk of cancer. Other studies suggest a protective effect for breast and lung cancer.

Selenium • Most studies of selenium have linked higher levels with a lower risk of cancer. Experiments in laboratory animals point out a protective effect against breast and colon cancer, in particular. One study, however, found that it enhanced skin and pancreatic tumors in some cases. Selenium is toxic in doses only slightly higher than the recommended amount of 50 to 200 micrograms.

Calcium • Studies seem to suggest a link between higher calcium intake and lower rates of intestinal cancer. In one recent study, men who ate more foods containing calcium and vitamin D (which helps the body absorb calcium) had about one-third the risk. There also is a theoretical link between higher calcium levels and lower rates of breast cancer, although this remains to be proven.

To make the "most wanted list," a food has to be extremely high in one of these factors believed to prevent cancer, a good source of several anticancer factors, or a low-fat substitute for a common high-fat diet item.

The Foods That Count

And now, here's a list of the 50 top anticancer foods, along with cooking tips to help maximize the protective power of each. The tips tell you how to prepare the foods in lower-fat ways, use them to replace high-fat items, or combine them with other foods on the list to make a super-protective dish.

Apricots • Rehydrate dried fruit in a small amount of warm apple or orange juice, add a little grated orange rind for extra flavor, if you like, then grind into a spread. Use on toast or muffins instead of butter, or as a low-fat crepe filling.

Bran Cereal • Use instead of low-fiber breakfast cereals as a crispy, fiber-rich topping for casseroles, or to coat chicken for baking. To "bread" chicken with bran cereal, dredge a boneless breast first in flour, then in egg white, and finally in crushed bran flakes.

Brazil Nuts • Crush and sprinkle on as a topping for casseroles and muffins.

Broccoli • Skip the butter sauce. Instead, steam, then dress broccoli (four servings) with a mixture of 1 teaspoon of corn oil or canola oil, 2 tablespoons lemon juice, and some tarragon or thyme to taste. Serve hot or chilled.

Brown Rice • To make a super salad, combine cooked rice with chopped carrots and red peppers and raisins. Dress with a light vinaigrette of canola oil and raspberry vinegar. Chill before using.

Brussels Sprouts • Forget the buttered bread crumbs. Instead, steam a pint of brussels sprouts, then marinate them along with some cherry tomatoes and mushrooms in a combination of 1 teaspoon of low-sodium soy sauce, 1 teaspoon of vegetable oil, 2 tablespoons of lemon juice, and 1 tablespoon of chopped parsley. Let stand for 30 minutes, then put them on skewers and broil for about 5 minutes.

Butternut Squash • Puree cooked squash and toss with pineapple chunks instead of butter.

Cabbage • For a crisp and sweet winter salad, toss shredded cabbage with raisins and apples. Top with an herb vinaigrette or a dressing made of whipped nonfat yogurt, celery seed, and honey.

Cantaloupe • To make a low-fat but creamy cooler, blend cantaloupe chunks with orange juice, nonfat yogurt, and crushed ice. Serve immediately.

Carrots • To give pureed carrots a buttery consistency without fat, steam carrot chunks with pear chunks, then puree together.

Cauliflower • Skip the cheese sauce. Steam and serve with a light tomato sauce seasoned with oregano and basil.

Chard • Boost the protective value of clear broth vegetable soups by adding chopped chard during cooking.

Chicken Breast • For a luscious and low-fat entree, brush skinless, boneless breasts with an apple cider/honey mixture and bake or broil. Baste frequently with the mixture during cooking.

Collard Greens • Use to replace bok choy in stir-fries. Or puree steamed collards with low-fat cottage cheese and use to stuff onions. Bake at 350°F for 30 to 40 minutes.

Corn Oil and Canola (Rapeseed) Oil • These mostly polyunsaturated and monounsaturated oils are rich sources of vitamin E. But since they're also fats, use them to replace (not in addition to) the butter, lard, or other saturated fat in your diet.

Evaporated Skim Milk • A boon to fat slashers. Use in place of cream in coffee, or whip and use immediately to top desserts. Flavor with a little maple syrup, if you like.

Figs (Dried) • To spice up brown rice, add $\frac{1}{4}$ cup chopped dried figs to 1 cup uncooked brown rice along with curry powder to taste. Cook the rice as usual.

Grapefruit • Make a great seafood salad of canned salmon, grapefruit sections and sliced cucumber. Drizzle with a dressing made of honey and citrus juices.

Great Northern Beans • Use beans to replace some of the meat in meat loaf. You'll boost the fiber and cut the fat. Use about 1 cup of chopped, cooked beans per pound of meat in your recipe.

Kale • For a delicious and moist fish dish, wrap fillets in steamed kale leaves and bake, basting frequently with chicken broth, until done.

Kidney Beans • For a zippy low-fat dip, blend 1 cup cooked kidney beans with chopped garlic, parsley, and scallions, and add chili powder to taste. Thin to desired consistency with tomato juice or water.

Kiwifruit • While usually used as a garnish, you can get more of the goodness of kiwis by simply cutting them in half and eating with a spoon.

Mangoes • Use chunks of mango in your favorite chutney recipe, then serve the chutney with meat, replacing fatty sauces and gravies.

Oatmeal • Instead of butter, use figs, apricots, prunes, and/or sunflower seeds to dress up your oatmeal and make it extra-protective.

Oranges • Combine chopped orange sections with a little honey and orange juice. Top fish fillets with the mixture and bake. They'll be moist and flavorful without butter.

Papaya • Puree ripe papaya into a sauce for poached chicken. Thin with a bit of water or fruit juice if necessary. Or combine pureed papaya with some nonfat yogurt and make frozen pops.

Peas (Edible-Podded) • Stuff with herbed, nonfat yogurt cheese (see listing for Yogurt Cheese-Nonfat).

Popcorn • Make in an air popper and season with your favorite herbs and spices instead of butter. Try adding chili powder for a savory snack, or honey, minced dried fruit, and minced nuts for a sweet one.

Potatoes • Mix nonfat yogurt or low-fat cottage cheese with dill, chives, and pepper (or other herbs) and use instead of sour cream to top baked potatoes.

Prunes • Make a nutrient- and fiber-packed compote: Mix prunes, raisins, apricots, grapefruit sections, and dried figs in a baking dish. Pour on enough orange juice to moisten and bake until warmed through, about 30 minutes.

Pumpkin • Update your pumpkin-pudding recipe for better health: Replace the whole milk with skim, and each egg with two egg whites. Add 2 or 3 tablespoons of dry milk powder to boost the calcium content.

Raisins • Sprinkle on salads to give them a sweet fiber lift.

Salmon (Canned) • Prepare a simple bisque by pureeing 1 can of salmon with 1 minced onion, $1\frac{1}{2}$–2 cups of stock, a dash of lemon juice, and $\frac{1}{2}$ cup of skim milk. Heat slowly until just simmering.

Sardines (Canned) • Look for sardines packed in mustard or tomato sauce instead of oil. Try a nutrient-dense sandwich of sardines in mustard sauce with spinach on crusty whole wheat bread.

Skim Milk • Simply substitute for whole milk and you reduce fat from over 48 percent of calories to less than 3 percent.

Spinach • Dress up a spinach salad with sliced strawberries and a vinaigrette of lemon juice, tarragon, vinegar, honey, grated lemon rind, and a small amount of oil.

Strawberries • Add pureed strawberries to applesauce for extra zip, as well as vitamin C and fiber.

Sunflower seeds • Toss seeds in low-sodium soy sauce, then toast at low heat in the oven or in a nonstick pan. Add to salads or yogurt.

Sweet Peppers • Roast some red peppers and cut them into strips. Toss with balsamic vinegar and a splash of olive oil for a tasty condiment.

Sweet Potatoes • Steam chunks of sweet potatoes with chopped dried apricots. Transfer to a baking dish, glaze with apricot nectar, and bake for about 20 minutes.

Swordfish • Add chunks of swordfish to stir-fries in place of beef. Broccoli and red peppers go well with it.

Tofu • Marinate in a small amount of low-sodium soy sauce mixed with oil. Stir-fry with vegetables.

Tuna (Canned) • Prepare a low-fat version of tuna salad by combining a can of drained, water-packed tuna with 1 tablespoon red wine vinegar and chopped onions to taste.

Turnips and Rutabagas • Mash with orange juice concentrate and a dash of cinnamon, instead of butter.

Wheat Germ • Dip fillets of white fish in egg white, then dredge in a mixture of toasted wheat germ, cornmeal, and Cajun spices before baking. They'll stay moist.

Whole Wheat Bread • To make a simple bread-pudding dessert, combine 4 cups bread cubes, two egg whites, 1½ cups skim milk, and a dash of cinnamon and nutmeg in a baking dish. Bake for 45 minutes at 350°F.

Yogurt (Nonfat) • Use as a substitute for sour cream in sauces. To keep it from curdling when heated, add 1 tablespoon cornstarch per cup.

Yogurt Cheese (Nonfat) • A great substitute for cream cheese in dips and spreads. The easiest way to make it: Use a coffee filter in a strainer positioned over a bowl. Pour nonfat yogurt into the filter and let drain (refrigerated) overnight. By morning the filter will contain yogurt cheese.

The Heart-Saver Diet Plan

Half of us have blood cholesterol levels over 200, enough to increase our risk for heart disease. Many of us have levels that exceed 250 or 300, putting us at very high risk. If only we had an easy solution to this cholesterol overload—a way to cut cholesterol quickly and safely.

Good news! Lately we've had dramatic confirmation that all this is within our reach. In fact, based on the latest ground-breaking research by James W. Anderson, M.D., of the University of Kentucky, and others, the evidence is clear: With the right dietary factors, it's possible to drop your blood cholesterol level 30 points in just 30 days! Granted, some of us may not experience such dramatic results. On the other hand, some of us may fare even better!

Your likelihood of dropping 30 points in 30 days depends on many individual factors, including your current cholesterol level. If your blood cholesterol is under 200 (considered a safe level), it probably won't drop much further.

The higher your blood cholesterol, however, the more it's likely to drop in response to these dietary changes. In other words, people who have the most to lose—those with the highest cholesterol readings—have the most to gain by following this program.

Magic Beans—and Oat Bran

The cornerstone of this cholesterol cure is soluble fiber. So called because it dissolves in water, soluble fiber (prevalent in oat bran and beans) is the star of the latest cholesterol-lowering research (*American Journal of Clinical Nutrition*).

In one study, for instance, Dr. Anderson's team studied 20 men, aged 34 to 66, with an average cholesterol level of 260. The men split into two groups. For three weeks, one group added 1½ cups of pinto and navy beans (cooked or in soup) to their daily diet. The other group added a cup of dry oat bran— served as hot cereal and in five muffins—each day.

The men's total cholesterol fell, on average, 60 points. LDL—low-density lipoprotein, the "bad" cholesterol known to cause heart disease—dropped 46 points (*American Journal of Clinical Nutrition*).

In another study, Dr. Anderson looked at ten men with cholesterol levels averaging 309 to see how oat bran and beans work in the long run. Six months into the study, the men's cholesterol had dropped an average of 76 points. Their LDL averaged 52 points lower.

In men who were monitored for two years, cholesterol and LDL had fallen slightly more. And HDL—high-density lipoprotein, the "good" cholesterol linked to heart health—had gained three points, another indicator of improved protection from heart disease (*Journal of the Canadian Dietetic Association*).

Although Dr. Anderson's studies were small and sometimes lacked a control group, he has duplicated his results many times.

What Makes Oat Bran and Beans Work?

Scientists know soluble fiber increases the output of bile (a digestive fluid made with cholesterol) in stool. They theorize the liver then has to make more bile, using more cholesterol. That leaves less cholesterol to circulate in blood and gum up arteries. Other theories hold that soluble fiber helps reduce the liver's cholesterol production. However they work, beans and oats generally do so with fewer side effects than cholesterol-lowering drugs, which can cause liver problems, constipation, and other complications. And lowering cholesterol with soluble fiber is less expensive than drug therapy, according to a recent study. For someone with cholesterol over 265, a year's supply of cholestyramine costs $1,442 and colestipol, $879. A year on oat bran, by comparison, costs only $248.

Here's one last reason to supplement your diet with oat bran and beans in preference to drug therapy: They taste good. Just whip up some of Dr. Anderson's recipes and taste for yourself.

So, what are you waiting for? Let's get started.

What to Do

To lower cholesterol permanently, you must stick with these dietary changes. And you're most likely to stick with changes you make slowly. That's why our four-week or 30-day program works so well. It's just enough time to ease into a healthy transformation. And it's enough time to register a significant (30-point) drop in your cholesterol reading. Now that's motivation!

Week One • Add about ⅓ cup of dry oat bran to your daily diet. You can get that amount in two oat-bran muffins (see recipe on page 67).

You'll need to drink lots of fluids—at least eight glasses a day. Fiber normally draws water into the intestine—that's how it softens stool. Without enough water, though, fiber sometimes blocks the intestine.

To round out the diet, Dr. Anderson recommends multivitamin and mineral supplements. There are two reasons. "First, many people may not get enough vitamins and minerals to begin with," says Dr. Anderson. "Second, since we don't know the long-term effects of fiber on vitamin and mineral absorption, we prescribe a supplement as a precaution." Take a daily supplement that delivers 100 percent of the Recommended Dietary Allowance.

Week Two • If your body has adjusted well to fiber so far, double your intake of soluble fiber. If you like oat bran, aim for ⅔ cup of oat bran per day. To get this amount, you need to eat four oat bran muffins or two muffins and ⅓ cup of oat bran cereal each day. (Just make sure you read the cereal labels; some are made with coconut oil, a saturated fat that raises cholesterol.)

If that sounds like a lot of oat bran, don't despair. You can meet your soluble fiber quota by eating beans. One cup of cooked beans contains the same amount of soluble fiber as ⅔ cup of oat bran. Better yet, eat oat bran and beans over the course of the day; two oat bran muffins for breakfast and a bowl of chili (containing $\frac{1}{2}$ cup of cooked beans) for lunch, for example, will easily fill the bill.

Afraid you'll get bored with this diet? Don't be. Legumes are among the most versatile of all foods. Try bean burritos or a hearty bean soup. Toss kidney beans in pasta salad. Puree garbanzo beans with pickles and low-fat dressing to make a delightful sandwich spread. Or stir-fry vegetables with firm tofu (made from soybeans). Dried or canned beans work just as well. Rinse canned beans before using, however, to reduce added salt.

Week Three • Continue with the recommendations for Week Two. And now, concentrate on trimming the fat from your diet. Like soluble fiber, a low-fat diet lowers cholesterol and promotes overall good health.

Defat the dairy products you eat. Choose low-fat and nonfat milk over whole, ditto for yogurt, and use evaporated skim milk instead of heavy cream or half-and-half. Avoid high-fat Cheddar and cream cheeses. Instead, try ricotta, mozzarella, and low-fat cottage cheese.

Limit your egg intake to two yolks a week. (Egg whites are fine; they don't contain any cholesterol.)

On sandwiches, hold the mayo—that is, the regular, high-fat kind. Light mayonnaise and mustard are better alternatives. On salads, use low-fat dressings.

For snacks, eat air-popped popcorn, pretzels, ginger-snaps, and vanilla wafers. And don't forget fruit—a good source of soluble fiber. Prunes, raisins, figs, dates, and apples are good choices, says Dr. Anderson.

Week Four • Continue with the recommendations for Week Three. Meanwhile, take the final steps to fine-tune your low-fat diet. First, eat fish—a healthy alternative to red meat—at least two times a week. Look to cold-water fish, such as mackerel, tuna, or salmon, which are rich in heart-healthy omega-3 fatty acids.

Second, select the leanest cuts of red meat, such as flank and tenderloin. Trim away all visible fat and remove skin from poultry. When possible, substitute poultry for red meat. In chili and lasagna, for instance, you can replace ground beef with ground turkey or chicken breast. Avoid fried foods; they're high in fat. When you must fry, "grease" the pan with a nonstick vegetable cooking spray.

Look to lean vegetarian dishes when you can. Think beans, of course, and pasta. Try whole wheat lasagna or spaghetti with a low-fat sauce as the centerpiece. "It's always better to get a red sauce than a cream sauce," says Dr. Anderson. "Fettuccine Alfredo is very high in fat. But fettuccine with marinara sauce is good.

"In general, try to cut down on beef and dairy products," says Dr. Anderson. "With these moderate changes, you can achieve a diet of less than 30 percent fat."

Finally, whenever possible, substitute olive and canola oils—loaded with cholesterol-cutting monounsaturated fat—for other fats.

All this wouldn't amount to a hill of beans—or oat bran—if Dr. Anderson's diet were hard to stick to. It isn't. His patients have followed the diet for up to seven years—maintaining low cholesterol all along.

Dr. Anderson's Oat Bran and Bean Recipes

Turkey Burgers

⅓ cup oat bran

1 pound lean ground turkey

Salt, pepper, and garlic powder, to taste

In a large bowl, mix enough oat bran with turkey so that the patties will hold their shape (you may not need all the oat bran). Mix seasonings in, then shape four patties.

Coat a heavy skillet with vegetable cooking spray. Cook patties over medium heat until they are done as desired.

Makes 4 patties

NOTE: From *Diabetes and Nutrition News,* James W. Anderson, M.D., editor.

Oat Bran-Raisin Muffins

2½ cups oat bran cereal

2 teaspoons brown sugar substitute

½ cup raisins

1 tablespoon baking powder

½ teaspoon salt

1 cup skim milk

4 ounces egg whites or egg substitute

1 tablespoon vegetable oil

Spray the bottoms only of a 10-cup muffin tin with vegetable spray or line with paper baking cups.

Preheat oven to 425°F.

In a large bowl, combine dry ingredients. Add milk, egg whites, and oil, and mix just until dry ingredients are moistened. Fill prepared muffin tin three-quarters full. Bake for 17 minutes or until golden brown.

Makes 10 muffins

NOTE: From the Specialized Diagnostic Treatment Unit, Veterans Administration Medical Center, Lexington, Kentucky.

Nine-Bean Soup

2 cups beans*

1 ham bone (1 pound)

1 large onion, chopped

1 clove garlic, chopped

2 bay leaves

1 can (16 ounces) tomatoes, cut into bite-size pieces

1 can (15 ounces) seasoned tomato sauce

$\frac{1}{2}$ teaspoon dried basil, if desired

$\frac{1}{2}$ teaspoon dried oregano, if desired

Wash and sort beans. Place in large Dutch oven with enough water to cover by 2 inches and soak overnight.

Drain beans; add ham bone, onions, garlic, bay leaves, and tomatoes. Cover and bring to a boil, then reduce heat and simmer for $1\frac{1}{2}$ to 2 hours, or until beans are tender.

Add tomato sauce and spices (if used). Simmer 30 minutes. Remove ham bone and bay leaves. Serve hot.

Makes 6 servings

*Any of the varieties of your choice, such as black beans, black-eyed peas, garbanzo beans, kidney beans, lentils, lima beans, mung beans, pinto beans, soybeans, split peas or white beans.

NOTE: From *Dr. Anderson's Life-Saving Diet,* by James W. Anderson, M.D. (Tucson, Arizona: The Body Press, 1986).

Chicken/Garbanzo Sandwich

1 can (8 ounces) garbanzo beans, drained and mashed

2 ounces cooked chicken, diced

$\frac{1}{2}$ cup minced carrots

2 teaspoons salad dressing

$\frac{1}{4}$ teaspoon salt, if desired

Dash each of pepper, ground sage, and ground allspice

4 slices whole wheat bread, or 2 pita rounds cut in half

Combine all ingredients except bread in a medium bowl. Mix thoroughly. Spread mixture on 2 bread slices; top with remaining slices and cut in half, or fill pita halves.

Makes 4 servings

NOTE: From *Dr. Anderson's Life-Saving Diet,* by James W. Anderson, M.D. (Tucson, Arizona: The Body Press, 1986).

Chili Con Carne

$\frac{1}{4}$ lb. lean ground beef, turkey, or chicken

$\frac{1}{2}$ cup chopped onion

1 clove garlic, minced

Ground cumin, to taste

1 can (16 ounces) kidney beans in tomato sauce

$\frac{1}{2}$ cup canned tomatoes and green chilies

In a medium saucepan, cook beef with onion, garlic, and cumin over medium heat until beef is browned, stirring to break up meat.

Add remaining ingredients. Bring to a boil, then reduce heat and simmer, uncovered, 10 minutes, stirring occasionally to blend flavors.

Makes 3 cups or 3 main-dish servings

NOTE: From *Dr. Anderson's Life-Saving Diet,* by James W. Anderson, M.D. (Tucson, Arizona: The Body Press, 1986).

Fighting Fire with Oil

By George L. Blackburn, M.D., Ph.D.

"Fire in the joints." That is what the word arthritis literally means—and what arthritis feels like—to millions of Americans.

The fiery pain is caused by inflammation, the common symptom of the two main kinds of arthritis. Osteoarthritis is a wear-and-tear disease that affects people as they age; bone cartilage wears down, triggering inflammation of the surrounding joint. Rheumatoid arthritis can strike young and old. It's a whole-body disease in which the immune system attacks the body's own tissues. Joint inflammation is just one symptom.

Although there is no cure for arthritis, a variety of medications are prescribed to alleviate the inflammation and pain, such as aspirin and ibuprofen. While these drugs are a boon to arthritis sufferers, they can have side effects. So it makes sense to get by with as little medication as possible.

One way to cut down on the need for medication may be to follow a diet that reduces inflammation. There is now scientific evidence that what you eat may make a difference in quenching the fires of both kinds of arthritis. (Just be sure to discuss any changes in diet or medication with your physician before taking action.)

EATING TO AVOID OSTEOARTHRITIS

Keeping your bones strong through proper nutrition may reduce your chances of developing osteoarthritis. Certain nutrients are crucial to bone health: calcium and vitamins C, D, B_6, and A. (There is no evidence, however, that rheumatoid arthritis can be prevented through dietary means.)

If you're eating a well-balanced diet, you're probably getting adequate amounts of these nutrients, with one exception: calcium. Many women don't consume enough of this mineral, especially if they avoid dairy products.

Women who are premenopausal should take in at least 1,000 milligrams of calcium a day. Postmenopausal women should consume about 1,200 milligrams. You may need a supplement to achieve these totals.

If you aren't sure whether your diet provides enough calcium—or any other nutrient—it's a good idea to write down everything you eat and drink for several days. Take your records to a dietitian for assessment.

Another way to help prevent osteoarthritis is to avoid obesity. Overweight increases the stress on weight-bearing joints. Shed excess pounds by eating a low-fat diet.

Fighting Fire with Fish Oil

The foods you eat—in particular, the forms of fat—may affect the level of inflammation, recent studies show.

The inflammation of arthritis is fed by certain prostaglandins, hormonelike substances that our bodies produce from fatty acids in the foods we eat. Most vegetable oils are rich in the class of fatty acids known as omega-6's, including linoleic acid and arachidonic acid. These fatty acids create the inflammatory prostaglandin called leukotriene. (Aspirin and other nonsteroidal anti-inflammatory drugs work by blocking the formation of leukotriene.)

But fish oil contains different fatty acids, the class known as omega-3's. In the body, omega-3 fatty acids compete with linoleic and arachidonic acid to create a different type of prostaglandin that doesn't trigger inflammation.

Studies of the effect of fish oil on people with arthritis seem to support this. In one study, for example, researchers examined the effects of fish oil on the symptoms of 33 patients with class 1, 2, or 3 rheumatoid arthritis. (There are four classes of rheumatoid arthritis, with class 1 being the mildest form.)

Before the study began, all the subjects endured morning stiffness for longer than 30 minutes and had multiple swollen and tender joints. For 14 weeks, half the group took 15 fish-oil supplement capsules a day, while the other half took placebos (harmless look-alikes); then the groups switched for another 14 weeks.

The results? When the people took fish oil, they experienced 33 percent less joint tenderness than when they took a placebo. They were also fatigue-free for over $2\frac{1}{2}$ hours longer each day (*Annals of Internal Medicine*).

Acting on the Evidence

There's no question that vegetable oils are generally beneficial to most people. Used instead of butter and lard, they can help lower cholesterol and reduce the risk of heart disease. But the results of this study and others like it suggest that people with arthritis may be a special case. I believe it may be worthwhile for them to try minimizing their intake of vegetable oils and maximizing their intake of oils rich in omega-3's.

Minimizing vegetable oils does not mean avoiding vegetables. It does mean cutting back on oil-containing products like salad dressings, fried foods, and margarine.

There are two good-guy vegetable oils that you can use, though, because they contain low levels of the omega-6's: canola oil, made from rapeseed, and olive oil. Simply use modest amounts of those oils in place of other vegetable oils in cooking. (Don't overdo the good-guy oils, though; for all-around good health, it's best to keep the overall level of fat in your diet to less than 30 percent of total calories.)

To get more omega-3's, make fish a regular part of your diet. In particular, look to the oil-rich, deepwater fish, such as salmon, tuna, halibut, and sardines (packed in water, not in vegetable oil).

There are other sources of omega-3's as well, most notably walnuts, soybeans, and tofu. But none deliver as much of this inflammation-fighting oil as deepwater fish do.

If you pay close attention to your diet, reducing vegetable oils and eating fresh or canned fish several times a week, you'll probably achieve good results without having to take fish-oil supplements.

But if changes in your diet don't seem to be helping, talk to a physician who is familiar with the studies on fish oil. He or she can guide you on proper supplementation, if it's appropriate.

Garlic Cloves Are Treasure Troves

Garlic, the "Stinking Rose," has been used and celebrated throughout history for its curative and culinary properties. First mentioned in Sanskrit as early as 5000 B.C., it has been heralded in the Bible and in the literature of the ancient Hebrews, Babylonians, Greeks, and Romans, and was a favorite fare of the ancient Egyptians, Vikings, and Phoenicians. Early pyramid builders were fed a daily ration of garlic for strength and endurance. The Greeks used it to cure snake bite and pneumonia.

During the Middle Ages, Europeans believed that garlic had the power to keep evil spirits out of their homes, and they adorned their doors with garlic braids and wreaths. The custom survives today—usually minus the superstition—in the garlic braids many cooks hang in their kitchens.

During World War I, garlic was successfully used to treat typhus and dysentery and to prevent infection and gangrene in battle wounds. Certain Slavic peoples still eat a clove of raw garlic with each meal during the winter months to prevent colds and flu.

Today in North America, people also celebrate garlic, but more for its culinary delights than for its traditional curative powers. Every summer, hundreds of thousands of people flock to the little town of Gilroy, California, near Monterey, the heartland of garlic growing, for the annual Garlic Festival. Festival-goers are treated to garlic everything—even garlic desserts.

While most people enjoy garlic's aromatic additions to cooking, are we ignoring the healing powers ancient peoples venerated? Are the medicinal uses of garlic valid, or are they just so much folklore—like using garlic as an aphrodisiac or to ward off vampires and evil spirits? The fact is, considerable evidence shows that garlic is a remarkable healer.

Scientific Validation

Most modern drugs were derived originally from plants. Garlic contains an amino acid derivative, alliin. When garlic is crushed or minced, an enzyme, allinase, is released, which converts the alliin to allicin, an antibiotic with antibacterial action equivalent to 1 percent penicillin. This antibacterial action validates the thousand-year-old tradition of using garlic to treat wounds and infections.

Most modern research regarding the medicinal properties of herbs, including garlic, has been conducted in Europe and Asia. Dozens of studies conducted at universities and hospitals in India, Japan, England, Poland, Russia, Canada, Germany, Romania, and elsewhere have established that garlic can lower serum cholesterol levels. In one study, people with high serum cholesterol who were given a garlic extract equivalent to about 10 grams of the herb per day for two months experienced a 28.5 percent reduction in cholesterol levels. In other studies, rabbits fed high-cholesterol diets who were given garlic had 1 to 80 percent lower blood cholesterol levels than the control group and 15 to 50 percent fewer atherosclerotic lesions. Although researchers aren't positive, they believe that garlic reduces serum cholesterol levels by somehow inhibiting its biosynthesis. Many believe that eating garlic regularly could have dramatic effects on artherosclerotic heart disease.

Garlic has also been shown to reduce blood pressure. Apparently garlic expands (dilates) blood vessel walls through the action of one of its components, methyl allyl trisulfide. Research has also shown that garlic thins the blood by inhibiting platelet aggregation, the tendency of blood cells to clump together. This reduces the risk of blood clots and may help prevent heart attacks.

In addition to its antibacterial properties and its beneficial effects on the circulatory system, studies have shown that garlic is also an antifungal agent. It appears to be effective against athlete's foot fungus, *Candida albicans,* the organism that causes most vaginal yeast infections, and at least 20 other pathogenic fungi. In a remarkable study conducted in China, 11 people suffering from cryptococcal meningitis, which is often fatal, were given garlic extract orally and garlic injections over a period of several weeks. All 11 garlic-treated patients recovered.

Garlic has been used as a cold and flu remedy for centuries. When the herb's allicin content was discovered, herbalists claimed that this antibacterial action explained garlic's traditional use for upper respiratory infections. However, colds and flu are caused by viruses, and antibiotics have no antiviral effects. Scientists attributed any cold and flu relief to garlic's pungent aroma, which acts as a mild decongestant, and to the fact that some people find garlic's aroma offensive, thus socially isolating cold and flu sufferers and limiting viral transmissions. Then in 1973, Japanese researchers showed that garlic is, in fact, able to prevent infection by influenza virus. Although this research was corroborated independently by researchers in Romania, the biochemical mechanism of this effect remains a mystery.

In addition to its medicinal properties, garlic is quite nutritious. It contains high levels of protein, vitamins A and C, thiamine, and trace minerals, including copper, zinc, iron, tin, calcium, potassium, aluminum, sulfur, germanium, and selenium.

So eat your garlic with glee, knowing that you're eating a delicious herb—an herb that also prevents illness.

What to Eat to Get Well Soon

By George L. Blackburn, M.D., Ph.D.

Remember the last time you were downed by a cold or an infection? Along with the sneezing or wheezing, the aches or the pains, you probably lost your appetite. Even your favorite foods seemed repugnant. "Eat, eat, you need your strength!" your spouse cajoled, your friends entreated. But for several days, you knew there was no way that you could get anything solid down the hatch—not anything that would stay down, that is.

What you were experiencing was the body's natural and ancient response to illness or shock. Through evolution, the body has become accustomed to lying down and resting when it's sick or injured. Your body doesn't want you to go about your usual activities, including eating. Instead, all its energy is concentrated on healing.

On the other hand, there is some truth to what your friends say: You do need proper nutrition for recovery. This dilemma is at the root of some confusing folklore: Feed a fever, starve a cold? Feed a cold, starve a fever? It's hard to keep straight!

But there are some simpler rules you can follow. The guiding principle is: Listen to your body.

If you're feeling hungry, that's terrific—by all means, eat. You need the nutrition.

If you don't feel like eating, then you should also listen to your body—for about five days. (People who are in poor health before their illness should follow a three-day rule, discussed below.) Usually the loss of appetite from a flu or cold virus or a local bacterial infection (such as a urinary tract infection) doesn't last much longer than five days. During those five days, let your appetite determine your food intake...and rest and let Mother Nature do her thing.

Fluids Are Essential

With any illness, however, there is one thing you must continue to put into your system: water. Keep yourself well hydrated, whether with water, juices, or broths. Liquids are especially important during viral infections.

As soon as you start to feel a little hungry, choose easily digestible, calorie- and nutrient-rich foods. The important nutrients for recuperation—vitamins A, C, B_6, and B_{12}, copper, magnesium, and zinc—are easy to get from most foods or from a standard multivitamin. If you can tolerate lactose, dairy foods are ideal when you're ill because they're high in nutrients and calories. Your pharmacy also sells medical foods, special nutrient-rich formulas, available without a prescription (brand names: Resource, Ensure, and Sustacal). They're easy to digest and contain all the key nutrients.

But if you still can't stomach anything after five days, that's when you must think about ignoring what your appetite is telling you. Prolonged fasting can harm your recovery. Let someone wave your favorite foods under your nose, and make yourself take a few bites.

If you can't possibly bring yourself to eat, tell your doctor. It could be a sign of a complication or secondary infection. Remember, nutrition is not on the mind of every physician. Your doctor may recommend supplements or a medical food after five days to ensure you're getting the nutrition you need.

Special Cases

Doctors have known for years that the shock of a broken bone can stop the function of your intestinal tract and your appetite. Again, this is the ancient signal that the body is in the acute phase of wound healing. The body wants to focus all its energy.

That loss of appetite from a broken bone can last for five to ten days. Often people lose a lot of weight after a broken bone, and if they're not eating properly, it can impair the bone healing. So the five-day rule applies here, too: After that period, try to stimulate your own appetite—and inform your physician if you're having problems.

The guidelines above are for people who were in good health before a temporary illness struck. Chronic illness is a different story. People who shouldn't wait five days to start eating include those who have been chronically ill, are underweight, or are very elderly. For them, a three-day (or less) rule is safer: After three days, start eating, even if it's just milk with a vitamin supplement or medical foods from your pharmacy. And again, if you're unsure and you find you're not hungry, consult your physician.

The Eight-Week Lower-Your-Blood-Pressure Plan

If you're one of the millions of Americans with high blood pressure, what's in your future? A lifetime of medication? Bland meals that make your taste buds scream for "just one pickle"? Never another glass of wine with dinner?

Not necessarily. Researchers have been hot on the trail of lifestyle "treatments" that can lower blood pressure without drugs and without taking the pleasure out of life. They say that if your diastolic pressure (the second number) is between 85 and 89 (high normal) or 90 and 104 (mild hypertension), you stand a good chance of lowering your blood pressure enough to get off medication entirely—or never having to start. The same goes if your systolic pressure (the first number) is 140 to 159 (borderline hypertension). And even if your numbers are higher, you may be able to cut way back on the drugs. All of this without embracing the austere existence of a monk.

The best of these nondrug approaches have been distilled into the following eight-week program. It's doctor-approved and based on the best and brightest antihypertension ideas from the scientific and medical communities.

The program goes slow and easy because sudden lifestyle changes hurt too much and rarely last. You phase in a few small changes each week, reinforcing or expanding them gradually. By the end of the eight weeks, you'll be safeguarding your heart and health in a dozen smart ways. And you'll have mastered a repertoire of blood-pressure-lowering techniques that can last you a lifetime.

A note before you begin: Hypertension is serious business. It increases your risk of stroke, heart disease, and kidney disease. So any blood-pressure program worth its sodium will start in your doctor's office, where the two of you can discuss your current diet, exercise level, physical condition, and medical history. Take this program along on your next office visit and go over it with your physician. Get his or her okay before making any changes. If you have pounds to lose, decide together on a realistic weight goal. Above all, take your medication faithfully until your doctor tells you to stop or cut back, and have your blood pressure monitored frequently.

Week 1

Start Taking 15-Minute Walks Three Times a Week • If you walk at a comfortable pace, you'll cover about ¾ mile each time. Exercise is step one in this program because it goes hand-in-hand with weight control—and, as hypertension experts point out, losing excess poundage is the surest nondrug technique for lowering blood pressure.

Drink Less. • Two alcoholic drinks a day, tops. (That's 24 ounces of beer, 8 ounces of wine, or 2 ounces of liquor.) More than that and you risk boosting your blood pressure. In fact, moderation in alcohol intake runs a close second to weight loss in sheer pressure-lowering power, experts say. Heavy drinkers who moderate or quit customarily enjoy a blood pressure drop of several points. Plus, if you're trying to lose weight, the empty calories don't help matters. So limit yourself or boycott booze entirely.

Tip: If you usually have wine with dinner, make a switch in substance—not ambiance. Pour chilled mineral water or salt-free seltzer into wine glasses, and add a twist of orange or lemon. Stow the bottle in an ice bucket!

Drink Milk Every Day • Or eat lots of broccoli. Or low-fat, low-sodium Swiss cheese. Or any combination of these and other foods that'll give you your daily ration of calcium (the Recommended Dietary Allowance, or RDA, is 800 milligrams per day). Research suggests that calcium not only works to keep bones stronger but may also help lower blood pressure in some people.

Tip: If consuming dairy products makes you feel bloated or gassy, you may be lactose intolerant. Try adding enzyme products like Lactaid and Lactrase (available in health-food stores) to milk before drinking. They break down the lactose (milk sugar). You can also buy lactose-reduced milk at some grocery stores.

Bonus Recipe:
High-Calcium Stir-Fry

2 large stalks broccoli

1 pound tofu*

  Minced garlic, to taste

  Peeled, minced gingerroot, to taste

1 tablespoon low-sodium soy sauce

2 teaspoons vegetable oil

2 cups cooked brown rice

In a wok or skillet, stir-fry broccoli, tofu, and seasonings in 2 teaspoons of vegetable oil. Season with soy sauce and serve hot over brown rice.

Makes 4 servings (319 calories, 485 milligrams of potassium, 215 milligrams of calcium, and 180 milligrams of sodium per serving)

*Tofu made with calcium sulfate has three times more calcium than nigari-prepared tofu.

Week 2

Increase Walking Time to 30 Minutes per Workout • You should cover about 1½ miles. If this pace is a strain, ease off until you get used to it.

Start Eating Fish Three Times a Week • Fresh or frozen, baked, broiled, or poached (but never fried), fish is a great catch. Its saturated fat content is usually low, and some fish (like salmon, mackerel, and tuna) score high in omega-3 fatty acids, which seem to have a beneficial effect on risk factors for heart disease. Flounder, cod, haddock, and fresh salmon are good sources of potassium, which has been linked to lower blood pressure and can be depleted by using diuretics.

Limit Yourself to One Serving of Either Cured Meat or Canned Soup per Week • Cured meats include bacon, sausage, hot dogs, and luncheon meats—all high-sodium and high-fat items.

Canned soups (unless they're labeled otherwise) also pack a lot of sodium. The problem with consuming too much sodium, of course, is that it can raise blood pressure in sodium-sensitive people. (Science hasn't yet devised a quick-and-easy test to tell who is and isn't sensitive.) Sodium consumption can actually work against many blood-pressure-lowering drugs.

"On the other hand," says Charles P. Tifft, M.D., associate professor of medicine at Boston University's Cardiovascular Institute, "restricting sodium to 2,300 milligrams per day—the amount found in 1 teaspoon of table salt (sodium chloride)—can lower blood pressure in one hypertensive out of three."

But say your blood pressure never does respond to sodium reduction. Should you feel free to salt up a storm? Sorry—experts think everybody should keep a lid on salt consumption.

Switch to Low-Fat Dairy Products • If you're drinking whole milk, go to 2 percent. If you're drinking 2 percent, try 1 percent. If you're a cheese lover, start enjoying only the low-fat (and low-sodium) varieties. Doing all this can make a big dent in your fat intake. And that can reduce your risk of heart disease and help you keep excess pounds off. After all, fat is loaded with calories—more calories per ounce than either protein or carbohydrates.

Week 3

Increase Your Walking Frequency to Five Days a Week • The more you exercise, the faster your metabolism works. The faster your metabolism, the more calories your body uses each day, which makes weight loss a whole lot easier.

Stop Adding Salt When You Cook • Don't add it even when you're boiling water for pasta. After a while, your taste buds may not even notice the difference.

Turn Your Thoughts to Fruit! • You don't have to give up dessert. Just don't equate dessert with high-sugar, high-fat goodies. Bananas, oranges, cantaloupe, and honeydew are all

82   *Diet Strategies That Heal*

potassium-rich, calorie-lean—and plenty sweet. Eating out?
Ask for a bowl of in-season fruits.

Bonus Recipe:
Cool and Fruity Dessert

1 peach, sliced

1 cup cantaloupe cubes

½ cup blueberries

1 tablespoon honey, warmed

1 tablespoon lime juice

½ cup low-fat yogurt

   Mint leaves, for garnish

In a medium bowl, mix peaches, cantaloupe, and blueberries.
In a separate container, blend honey, lime juice, and yogurt.
Serve fruit mixture in individual dishes and top with yogurt
sauce. Garnish with mint leaves.

*Makes 2 servings (138 calories, 512 milligrams of potassium,
118 milligrams of calcium, and 50 milligrams of sodium per
serving)*

Week 4

Switch to Even Leaner Milk • If you're drinking 2 percent, try
1 percent. If you're on 1 percent, drink skim. Surprise: One cup
of skim milk contains 406 milligrams of potassium (even more
than fattier milks), 301 milligrams of calcium, and 127 milligrams of sodium.

Stop Salting Your Food at Mealtime • Instead, fill your salt
shaker with your favorite herbs or a no-sodium seasoning and
shake away.

Discover the Potato! • At least three times a week, have a
baked spud or make a potato-based dish. Potatoes are fat free
and loaded with potassium.

Bonus Recipe: Tomato/Potato Salad

1 pound new potatoes, halved

1 pound tomatoes, cut into chunks

¼ cup minced fresh basil

2 teaspoons olive oil

In a large saucepan, steam potatoes until tender, about 8 to 10 minutes. Place in a large bowl and immediately toss with tomatoes, basil, and olive oil. Serve at once, while still warm.

Makes 4 servings (123 calories, 736 milligrams of potassium, and 18 milligrams of sodium per serving)

Week 5

Pick Up the Pace • Aim to cover 2 miles in a half hour if you can do so without strain. You should feel energized by your walks—aches or excessive tiredness are signals to ease up a bit.

Take 10 Minutes and Relax • Every day. And we don't mean lie down and worry about tomorrow's workload. But try some serious relaxing by using definite techniques, such as progressive muscle relaxation, meditation, and biofeedback. Research suggests that in some people, these may have a modest, long-term lowering effect on blood pressure.

Week 6

Move beyond Walking • Now's the time to start spicing up your workouts with a little variety—your hedge against exercise boredom and burnout. One or two days a week, skip your walk and swim a few laps at your local pool instead. Or bike around the block. Or whatever. To start, put in about 15 minutes on each new exercise session and slowly work up to 30 minutes, if you can. Don't push and don't overload. You should still be active five days a week.

Be aware, though, that some doctors do not recommend weight machines and weight lifting for hypertensives because they may raise rather than lower blood pressure.

Get into Low-Sodium Snacking • Ban salty snack foods, such as potato chips, pretzels, and nachos, from your diet. Instead, nosh on unsalted air-popped popcorn, unsalted pretzels, rice cakes, melba toast, or carrots. (Caution: Low-sodium potato and corn chips are high in fat.)

Say Yes to Yogurt! • And say it three times a week. Plain and simple, yogurt boosts your calcium intake—one low-fat cup dishes out 414 milligrams (that's over half the RDA); spoon up 8 ounces of nonfat and you get 452! Plenty of potassium, too.

Yogurt subs beautifully for fatty no-no's like cream, sour cream, and oil. Browse through low-fat cookbooks for yogurt-based salad dressings, soups, dips, and drinks.

Bonus Recipe: Honey/Berry Frozen Yogurt Pops

1 pint fresh strawberries

⅓ cup honey

1 teaspoon vanilla extract

2 cups low-fat yogurt

Place berries in blender or food processor and blend until smooth. Add honey (use less if berries are very sweet), vanilla, and yogurt. Blend again.

Pour mixture into ice-pop molds or ice-cube trays, cover with plastic or foil, and freeze for 1 hour, then place wooden sticks in molds. Freeze until solid.

Makes about 1 quart, or 8 ½-cup molds (92 calories, 202 milligrams of potassium, 110 milligrams of calcium, and 41 milligrams of sodium per serving)

Week 7

Cut Out Cured Meats Entirely • Instead, go for lean cuts of beef, pork, and lamb, along with turkey and chicken. They usually contain less fat and sodium.

Fill Up on Veggies, Three to Four Servings a Day • Buy them fresh or frozen, or look for the reduced-sodium canned variety. Steam or bake or microwave or stir-fry—easy on the oil! Once a week, take a bean to lunch. You probably know that beans are a high-fiber, high-protein food. But did you know that they're also high in potassium?

Did you know that some canned beans can have less potassium and more than 100 times more sodium than the beans you buy dried and cook yourself? Enough said.

Bonus Recipe: Three-Bean Salad

1 cup white marrow beans

1 cup red kidney beans

1 cup fresh green beans, cut into 1-inch pieces

1½ tablespoons olive oil

3 tablespoons red wine vinegar

2 cloves garlic, minced

¼ teaspoon dried oregano

½ teaspoon black pepper

1 large onion, sliced and separated into rings

2 stalks celery, thinly sliced

2 tablespoons minced parsley

In a large saucepan, cook the marrow beans and kidney beans, then drain. Place in a large bowl and set aside.

In a medium saucepan, steam green beans for 5 minutes. Add to bowl and set aside.

In a small bowl, mix olive oil, vinegar, garlic, oregano, and pepper. Pour mixture over beans and chill overnight. Before serving, add onion, celery, and parsley. Toss and serve on romaine or other lettuce leaves.

Makes 6 servings (131 calories, 463 milligrams of potassium, 46 milligrams of magnesium, 67 milligrams of calcium, and 18 milligrams of sodium per serving)

Week 8

Lengthen Your Walks to 45 Minutes a Day • Cover 2 to 3 miles each time. Continue to substitute other kinds of workouts once in a while. Keep on movin'!

Weigh Yourself • By exercising and following our low-fat, low-salt suggestions, you've probably dropped a few pounds by now—without counting a single calorie. Although a 10-pound loss may produce a drop in blood pressure, it usually takes 20 pounds to make a noticeable difference. Of course, you're best off at your goal weight.

If you have much further to go, talk to your doctor about a long-range weight-loss plan. You may decide to join a support group; self-help organizations can put you on the road to permanent weight loss.

Evaluate Your Overall Progress • Now how's your blood pressure? Has your doctor reduced your medication? Are you successfully limiting alcohol and sodium? You may need longer to get some changes in place; don't give up. Continue to consult with your doctor as you work toward lower blood pressure—and better health!

WEEK 9 AND BEYOND

Once you have completed the eight-week program outlined in the chapter, there are still some things you should do to maintain your new, healthy lifestyle.

Every Day

• Take your blood pressure medication, if any.
• Make food choices in line with reaching or maintaining your weight goal.
• Drink less alcohol or none at all. If you do indulge, stop after two drinks.
• Drink milk or eat calcium-rich foods to get your RDA of calcium.

(continued)

WEEK 9 AND BEYOND—*Continued*

- Stick to low-fat or nonfat dairy products.
- Limit your intake of sodium to 2,300 milligrams.
- Eat plenty of fresh fruits and three to four servings of vegetables, including leafy greens and broccoli.
- Take a 10-minute relaxation break.

Five Times a Week (at least)

- Exercise.

Three Times a Week (at least)

- Eat fish.
- Enjoy low-fat, nutritious foods, such as potatoes, yogurt, and whole grains such as brown rice and whole wheat pasta.

Once a Week (at least)

- Eat some beans.

Occasionally

- Weigh yourself.
- Order a sinful dessert.

Beat Breast Cancer with Low-Fat Fare

By George L. Blackburn, M.D., Ph.D.

Can a low-fat diet protect against breast cancer? It's an important question, since 1 out of 11 American women develop the much-feared disease.

Unfortunately, the National Cancer Institute (NCI) canceled a major study (funded by our tax dollars) that might have answered that question once and for all. The Women's Health Trial would have involved some 32,000 women between the ages of 45 and 69. Half of them would have been put on a low-fat diet (consuming about 20 percent of their daily calories from fat), and the other half would have continued to consume the typical high-fat American diet (nearly 40 percent of calories from fat). The researchers planned to follow the women's health for ten years, to see if a low-fat diet could significantly reduce breast-cancer incidence in middle-aged and older women.

Those results would have been tremendously useful; I'm personally very disappointed by the NCI's decision. At the same time, there's no reason for women to wait for the final verdict before taking action toward adopting a low-fat diet. The evidence to date may not be conclusive but, in my view, it is too strong to ignore. The Surgeon General's new *Report on Nutrition and Health* emphasizes the reduction of dietary fat intake.

The Case against Fat

There's a broad consensus in the scientific community that eating a low-fat diet decreases the initiation and the progression of many cancers. Scientists aren't certain why. But we do know that fats can impact the functioning of the immune response, and fatty acids can directly activate tumor-cell growth.

In terms of breast cancer, many studies do suggest that a high-fat diet—and obesity—increase the risk. For example:

• When animals eat a low-fat diet (about 5 percent of calories from fat), they experience one-third to one-quarter the breast tumors of animals on higher-fat diets (about 20 percent of calories from fat).
• We know that fat tissue in the body produces hormones similar to those produced by the ovaries. And researchers have documented that sex hormones stimulate the growth of breast cancer (women whose ovaries are removed prior to age 37 have less breast cancer later in life). Presumably, a lean body is less likely to produce high levels of these cancer-promoting hormones.
• Cross-cultural studies have found that people whose diets

are the lowest in fat have the lowest breast-cancer rates. In Japan, for example, the breast-cancer rate is 4 per 100,000 women per year; in the United States, the level is more than double that—9 cancers per 100,000 women per year. The rice-and-fish-nibbling Japanese consume roughly 20 percent of their calories from fat, about half the fat intake of steak-and-fries-gobbling Americans.

• In related studies, researchers have found that breast cancer rates among Americans of Japanese descent are much higher than the rates of their Japanese cousins. In one such study, researchers found that, among the grandchildren of Japanese who immigrated to Hawaii, the incidence of breast cancer was as high as that of Hawaiian Caucasians. That suggests the American diet, not genetics, may be at fault.

Fat or Calories?

The U.S. Department of Agriculture recommends that we cut our fat intake as part of their guidelines for healthy eating. So why aren't doctors advising women—particularly those with a family history of cancer—to reduce their fat intake?

One reason is the ongoing, confusing debate in scientific circles about whether it's the fat intake or the calorie intake that affects cancer risk. Some scientists maintain the reason women in countries like Japan get less cancer is not because they eat less fat than we do but because they take in fewer calories.

My view is that, for practical purposes, it really doesn't matter whether it's the fat or the calories that affects cancer risk more. When you switch from a high-fat to a low-fat diet, you can't help but eat fewer calories. So you accomplish both goals . . . and more!

A low-fat diet—if done properly, by upping your intake of grains, fruits, and vegetables—also increases the proportion of cancer-fighting fiber and nutrients that you consume.

The final bonus: On a low-fat, low-calorie diet, weight drops, and low body weight is another protective factor against cancer.

How Low Should You Go?

Another reason that doctors resist making the low-fat prescription is because of indications that for a low-fat diet to be effective against breast cancer, it should be very low in fat—even below the standard 30 percent of calories recommended by the NCI and others.

This is a very controversial point. One major study that raised the issue was the Harvard Nurses Study, conducted by Walter Willett, M.D., and associates at the Harvard Medical School. The researchers collected data on the eating habits and breast cancer rates of 89,000 nurses, aged 34 to 59. The women were classified in four groups, according to their fat intake. In the "low-fat" group, the mean fat intake was 32 percent of calories from fat, while in the "high-fat" group, the mean fat intake was 44 percent of calories from fat.

On first glance, it appears that the study disproved the fat/breast cancer link: Over a period of four years, the researchers found that the nurses in the low-fat group had as great a chance of developing breast cancer as those who ate more fat.

The question that comes to mind, however, is whether the low-fat diet was low enough. All the nurses ate more than 30 percent of calories from fat, while the cross-cultural evidence clearly suggests you need to reduce your fat intake to 20 percent to benefit.

Dietary Goals to Prevent Breast Cancer

The development of cancer is a 25-year proposition. So clearly, a low-fat diet is important even for girls in grade school and high school, to reduce the risk of cancer later in life. In my view, a diet that contains less than 30 percent of calories from fat would be a prudent goal for girls, as well as for women under 50 who are not at a heightened risk for breast cancer.

I believe that women over 50 and women at high risk for breast cancer (because of family or personal history) would do well to cut back even further. Their goal should be to eat a diet that contains about 20 percent of calories from fat.

Even if early breast cancers have begun, there is still time to lower fat, restrict calories, and eliminate obesity, to slow the growth and progression of a tumor. (Keep in mind that a low-fat diet should not be considered a substitute for medical treatment. Also, we do not recommend that women undergoing chemotherapy for breast cancer or with advanced breast cancer attempt to begin a low-fat diet; all dietary therapy must be coordinated with an oncologist.)

Preventing Recurrences

Can a low-fat diet help prevent recurrences of breast cancer in women who've had mastectomies? We may have an answer to that question in a few years. Although the NCI canceled the Women's Health Trial, it is now sponsoring a small study, WINS (Women's Intervention Nutrition Study), which will involve about 300 women across the country who have had partial mastectomies. Immediately after surgery, half the women will receive the drug tamoxifen, which blocks estrogen; the other half will receive the drug and go on a low-fat diet. Which group will experience more recurrences of breast cancer? We're just enrolling women for the study now, and the results won't be known for four years. It will be an important test of the low-fat diet in delaying or preventing the recurrence of breast cancer in women over 50.

Finally, it's important to remember that a low-fat diet is just one part of a total cancer-prevention plan that should include monthly self-exams and regular mammograms if you're in a high-risk category. Consult your doctor or your local chapter of the American Cancer Society for more information.

WHAT IT TAKES TO CUT THE FAT

A low-fat, calorie-restricted diet isn't easy in the beginning, but with a little instruction, you'll find that it's not so difficult.

It does involve counting—but instead of calories, you'll be counting grams of fat, every day. Your total calorie intake, and body weight, should fall naturally as you eat less fat.

Set Your Fat Goal

It's best to get a professional nutritionist's guidance, but here's how to figure out, roughly, how many grams of fat you should be eating each day:

1. Start by calculating how many calories you eat, or should eat, in a day. You can estimate your target daily calories by multiplying your desired weight by 12. (This level may sound low compared to other recommendations you've read, but remember: Restricted calorie intake can protect against cancer.)

2. Next, multiply that figure by 0.2—since 20 percent of calories should be from fat. If your goal is 30 percent of calories from fat, multiply by 0.3.

3. Then, divide that figure by 9 (the number of calories in a gram of fat).

Let's say, for example, that your goal is to reduce your fat intake to 20 percent of total calories. Your ideal weight is 130 pounds. To arrive at your target daily fat count (in grams), first multiply 130 (your ideal weight) by 12 for a desired daily calorie count of 1,560. Next, multiply 1,560 by 0.2 (if you want to consume 20 percent of calories from fat) for a daily intake in fat calories of 312. Then divide 312 by 9, to arrive at your goal of 35 fat grams per day.

These are average figures for a woman 5'4" to 5'6" tall. Keep in mind that, if you are shorter than that or are extremely active, your calorie requirements may differ. Consult with a professional nutritionist for a tailor-made plan.

(continued)

WHAT IT TAKES TO CUT THE FAT—
Continued

Count the Grams

The next step is to learn to stick to your goal by counting fat grams, food by food, and by keeping a daily tally. You can purchase a book that lists the fat contents of various foods.

Fast foods are a Pandora's box of fat. One fried-chicken sandwich or deluxe cheeseburger at a fast-food joint can contain nearly 50 grams of fat—more than twice what the typical woman should be eating a day!

Read labels, too. What you read may amaze you. A cup of unbuttered noodles provides only a gram of fat, but a cup of fried rice contains 15 grams, which could be half your daily allotment. Sherbet contains only 4 grams of fat, compared to 24 grams in a cup of ice cream. A pat of butter, by the way, contains about 4 grams of fat, and an egg about 6 grams.

How can you tell if you're following a low-fat diet correctly? One good sign is if you lose a little weight. Even people who aren't obviously overweight, and who switch to a low-fat diet, often lose about 5 pounds in the first three months. Some people lose less, and overweight people may lose much more. Also, your blood cholesterol (determined by taking an average value of two or three finger-stick blood tests) decreases, since dietary fat is a major cause of high cholesterol.

Weight-Loss Updates

Gear Up Your Mind and Get Thin

Let's face it. Your body really doesn't mind running on a few less calories a day. For that matter, it even thrives on your daily workout. So if the whole business of weight loss is okay with your body, where do a lot of the problems occur? With your mind.

To psych yourself slim, you must readjust both your weight-loss program and your attitude. Results will be much better and come with a lot less stress. Here are a few dos and don'ts.

1. *Do* take a few minutes to look back over your past weight-loss attempts. "Many people tend to try the same techniques over and over again even though the techniques don't work," says Linda Crawford, program specialist for Green Mountain at Fox Run, a residential program for weight and health management in Ludlow, Vermont. "They get into a mind-set that says the problem is not with the technique but with themselves. This might not be the case at all. Techniques that may be perfectly suited to the personalities of some people are inherently not useful to others." Check for the breakdown point in your last weight-loss attempt, see what caused it, and leave that technique out of your new game plan.

2. *Don't* try to change too many behavior patterns at once. "When you first start your weight-management program, there is the tendency to try changing your whole life in one fell swoop," says Crawford. "This only creates incredible stress, which sets you up for a fall. What you want to do is isolate and change little behavior patterns, things that you can accomplish with a fair chance of success. For example, start off the first week by no longer snacking in the car. When you've got that down, throw in a boycott of food in front of the TV. As you get one small section of your life under control, go on to the next."

3. *Do* a little homework into the biology of weight loss. "The first thing we do when people come to us is show them exactly what it takes to lose a pound of fat," says Patrick O'Neil, Ph.D., of the Weight Management Center of the Medical University of South Carolina. "The bottom line is that to lose a pound of fat, you need to burn up 3,500 calories over and above what you take in. People who don't realize this tend to become disappointed when they aren't losing a pound a day, even though that kind of fat loss is next to impossible. They may give up, despite the fact that they were actually doing quite well." Tip: Find out what your physician thinks is a reasonable weight-loss schedule for you. Believe it or not, it might be a little more lenient than the one you cooked up on your own.

4. *Don't* subscribe to "all or none" thinking. "Many people trying to lose weight are unduly harsh on themselves," says Dr. O'Neil. "They assume that if they aren't doing everything in their weight-loss plan with total perfection, then they are failing and might as well give up. This kind of thinking guarantees failure because no one is perfect. Everyone deviates from their weight-loss plan at some point. The trick is to adopt 'matter of degree' thinking, where you evaluate yourself as being 98 percent on target or 85 percent and so on." Keep in mind that if you blow your diet as much as one-fifth of the time, that's still an 80 percent success rate, which on a grading scale of A to F would give you a B—certainly no reason to drop out!

5. *Do* start planning your days with the same precision as an executive. "A lot of eating is done as a transitional activity between engagements," says Crawford. "You may be out shopping and sit down to have a Danish and coffee. Or you come home from work, drop your things, and have a little snack before walking the dog.

"Instead, you want to look for those little interludes during the day and find activities to fill them up." Instead of coming home and eating right away, walk the dog, change your clothes, read the mail, and watch the evening news. By the time you're done, it's dinnertime. If you need a break from shopping, take a walk around the outside of the mall or take along a book to read on a bench or in your car if there's nowhere to sit in the shopping area.

6. *Don't* go out and buy a bikini or suit four sizes too slim. "I've never seen this motivational technique work," says Crawford. "What ends up happening is you keep trying the clothes on too soon. When they don't fit, you're reminded that things aren't moving along as fast as you'd like. Then the whole project starts to look impossible, and you give up." What she suggests is that you cut out a picture of that swimsuit or dress and put it on the refrigerator as a gentle reminder of what you'd like to be wearing next year at this time.

7. *Do* get yourself a hobby. "There is no doubt about it, eating is one of the more enjoyable things in life," admits Dr. O'Neil. "So if you're going to cut down on it, you're also going to need a substitute, something to reward yourself with." This could mean going to the movies a little more than usual, taking up hang-gliding, or collecting coins. But make it something you can truly get lost in, something that, for a time, lets you forget the world around you.

8. *Don't* make your end goal your only goal. "If your final goal is the only thing you have in your sights, it's going to look like a long row to hoe," says Crawford. "You want to avoid thinking that maybe the row is too long and you might as well give up. The way around this is to set up a series of smaller goals and rewards." Plan on rewarding yourself after every 2, 3, or 5 pounds, and make those rewards progressively more grand as you go along. Save the trip to Europe as a reward for making it to the last goal.

9. *Do* gear up for action. "Get yourself some bright, exciting exercise clothes," suggests Crawford. "They make your mind say, 'I'm going to put them on, I'm going to get ready, and I'm going to feel good about doing this.' "

10. *Do* keep a good supply of humor material on hand. When chocolate-eclair deprivation leaves you a little blue, administer a dose of the Marx brothers. A couple of laughs will put everything, including your diet, in a better light.

The Key to Big-Time Weight Loss

So you want to lose a whole lot of weight—30, 40, 50, 100 pounds or more!

Don't let the prospect overwhelm you. The truth is, you can lose as much weight as you want to. It won't be easy. It takes a lot of time and commitment. But with this new plan— and your determination—you'll shed pounds at a safe and steady pace. Without drugs and without fasting, you'll chalk up *big* losses that last. And just think of the energy, health, and confidence you'll gain!

Laying the Groundwork for Success

Losing weight requires changing long-standing habits. And if you're a big person, chances are you'll need to make big changes. That takes continuous effort and motivation. "If you're not really motivated, you'll keep losing weight and gaining it back," says Susan Ross, Ed.D., a registered dietitian and weight-loss researcher at the College of DuPage, in Glen Ellyn, Illinois. "And that's not healthy. Don't try to lose weight until you're ready."

To see if you've got what it takes to succeed, ask yourself the following questions.

Why Do I Want to Lose the Weight? • You should have compelling, personal, and positive reasons. If it's because your spouse is nagging you, you'll probably start resenting your sacrifices, especially if the bickering doesn't go away. Is it because you hate your fat self? Too bad, because hate doesn't motivate—it just makes you feel bad. Don't bother trying to lose weight on a whim either. A whim is hardly enough to withstand the power of ice cream sundaes and pizza.

Another tip: "Never try to use weight loss to solve problems that are not weight related," advises Barbara Jacobson, Ph.D., a psychologist and coauthor with her husband, Richard Stuart, Ph.D., of *Weight, Sex and Marriage: A Delicate Balance*. If you think being thin will magically cure all your problems, you'll be pretty disappointed when you finally get there.

So what's a good reason?

In one study, successful weight-losers (those who lost 30 or more pounds and kept it off for a year) had their own custom-tailored incentives. "Everyone said, 'This time I knew I had to do it for myself. Not for others, not for a special occasion, but for myself,' " says Ross, who conducted the research. "They said they had to do a little soul-searching. Some had reasons attached to midlife. They realized they couldn't do anything about getting old, but they could do something to improve the quality of life."

Will I Succeed? • Only if you can answer yes, without hesitation, are you ready to take on the challenge. "If you don't believe you can lose weight, you probably won't," says Maurice Larocque, M.D., president of the Canadian Society of Bariatric Physicians and author of *Be Thin through Motivation*. "If you make a mistake, you might say, 'I knew I couldn't do it,' and you'll probably stop trying."

"One of the worst problems I see in people who are trying to lose a lot of weight is that many of them have tried to lose weight unsuccessfully in the past, and they have a failure mentality," says Joyce D. Nash, Ph.D., author of *Maximize Your Body Potential*. "And that can be a self-fulfilling prophecy."

The fact is, you can do it this time if you want.

"Think of changes in your job or family life in which you've successfully gained new knowledge or skills," suggests Ross. "Weight loss and maintenance are just another change in day-to-day life that can be coped with and mastered."

Do I Need to Be Fat? • That may sound like a silly question. But when Dr. Jacobson and Dr. Stuart surveyed 25,000 women, they were amazed at the number of them who described the usefulness of being fat and the pitfalls of being thin. These women said they wanted to lose weight. But unconsciously, they weren't so sure. And their mixed feelings sabotaged their diet efforts.

Fat can be a handy excuse to avoid risking failure or rejection. "Some overweight women won't try to improve their lives—for instance, get a new job or start a new hobby—until they've lost a sufficient amount of weight," says Dr. Jacobson. "But they never lose enough to take that first step. Losing weight would rob such a person of her major excuse for clinging to the security of her home."

The real problem may be that you're afraid to take risks to achieve your wishes. If you're thinking about making a move to better your life, do it now. Then concentrate on losing weight.

When to See a Doctor

Assuming all the indicators say you're ready to lose (and you have a lot to lose), your next step should be to your physician for a physical. This is a necessary precaution, since carrying around that excess baggage—and losing it—can create its own set of health problems. You need to know your limitations.

For added assurance, schedule a follow-up appointment after you've shed 30 pounds. If you're taking medication for such problems as high blood pressure or diabetes, you may require an adjustment in the dosage as you lose weight.

HURDLE #1:
YOU'RE HAUNTED BY CRAVINGS

You may believe the urge to eat will get worse and worse until you douse it with a hefty serving of chocolate.

"But actually, gratifying an urge by eating makes urges stronger and more frequent," says G. Alan Marlatt, Ph.D., director of the Addictive Behavior Research Center at the University of Washington, Seattle. "In contrast, letting the urge pass will weaken it. If you can outlast enough of the urges, they will fade to obscurity."

Just so you don't feel deprived (thinking of life without chocolate is too much for a person to bear), plan to treat yourself every once in a while—say, once a week.

Calorie Cuts for Optimum Weight Loss

Now you're ready to tackle the *big* issue: how to budge 30-plus pounds from your frame. Surprise: The answer is not "starve yourself." Crash diets are self-defeating. Your body's natural response to starvation is to slow its metabolic rate. So even though you're eating fewer calories, your body's caloric requirements have dropped proportionately. "This makes it increasingly difficult to continue losing weight and much easier to gain it back," says weight-loss expert George Blackburn, M.D., Ph.D.

The key to losing a lot of weight is to eat enough to keep your metabolism charged but less than you'd need to maintain that excess weight. The arithmetic is simple: If you're 30 to 100 pounds overweight, cut your daily intake by just 500 calories; if you're 100-plus pounds overweight, you can afford to cut your daily intake by 1,000 calories. The trick is to choose the right kind of calories to cut.

You could take an arbitrary 500 calories from your daily diet with good results. But for more efficient weight loss, identify the high-fat foods you eat—the buttery muffins, croissants, grilled cheese sandwiches, cheeseburgers, blue cheese dressings, mayonnaise-laden sandwiches, chocolate bars, and other foods—and, each day, give 500 calories' worth the ax (or 1,000, depending on how much you have to lose). Remember, of course, if you're replacing a high-fat food (such as a cheeseburger at 335 calories) with a lower-fat item (such as a turkey breast sandwich at 281 calories), you'll have to calculate (335-281 = 54 calories) exactly how much that substitution contributes to your daily calorie-reduction goal. To do this, you will need a calorie-counting chart, preferably one that lists the fat content of foods.

Fat calories, as we've been saying for some time, count more than calories from carbohydrates. They are readily stored as body fat, whereas carbohydrate calories have to be converted to fat—a process that burns calories. By reducing your intake of high-fat foods by 500 or 1,000 calories, then, you can maintain a metabolic edge and maximize your weight-lowering potential.

Cutting Down without Giving Up

"You probably already know what's fattening and what's not," says Susan Olson, Ph.D., director of psychological services at Southwest Bariatric Nutrition Center, in Scottsdale, Arizona, and author of *Keeping It Off*. "The trouble is, too

---

HURDLE #2:
YOUR MOTIVATION FALTERS

Are you starting to see your weight-control program as a nasty, horrible burden you must bear? Take a minute to write down everything that's interfering with your plans. Has bad weather curtailed your morning walks? Does dining out tempt you with fattening fare?

Consider each of these obstacles a minichallenge. Check out a shopping mall as an alternative trail, for example. Choose ethnic restaurants with a wide variety of low-fat foods.

Don't give up. Just use your imagination to come up with creative solutions.

often the foods we need to give up are the ones we relish the most.

"I start treatment by asking my clients what they're not willing to change. If someone's not willing to give up chocolate, she'll fail at any diet that prohibits it. So we negotiate what she is and is not willing to do. Maybe she'll decide to eat chocolate three times a week instead of every day. Or maybe she's able to cut out enough other fatty foods so she can 'afford' the daily candy bar."

You can cut out fat calories with minimum pain if you use a few portion-control techniques.

If you have the tendency to finish the whole carton of ice cream, try buying a single-serving ice cream bar instead. Do you go back for seconds and thirds at dinner? Then wrap up the leftovers and freeze them before you have a chance to mindlessly eat more.

Eat slowly (spend at least 20 minutes on your meal) and you'll feel full with less food. That's because it takes 20 to 30 minutes after you start eating for your body's "feel-full" hormones to kick in. If you eat too fast, you won't feel too stuffed until it's too late.

Easy Exercise:
The Other Half of the Weight-Loss Equation

The heavier you are, the harder exercise will be. But the more you weigh, the more you can benefit from exercise, too. Exercise, together with a diet moderately reduced in fat calories, can get your metabolism in high gear.

The experts' recommendation? Walking. It's gentle on the joints and burns more fat than the high-impact kind of exercise. (A 1-mile brisk walk is worth about 100 calories.)

Just start slowly and take it at your own pace. Put petroleum jelly or talcum on your thighs to cut down on chafing. "If you're extra heavy, you may need the extra support of a running shoe instead of a walking shoe," says Steven I. Subotnick, D.P.M., a sports podiatrist from Hayward, California.

HURDLE #3:
YOU HIT A PLATEAU

Plateaus can be devastating and discouraging. After all your work, the scale refuses to budge! Maybe it even inches back up ever so slightly.

Don't panic. Plateaus are totally natural. "In general, heavier people may lose weight more rapidly at first, but the weight comes off slower as they get closer to their ideal weight," says Garth Fischer, Ph.D., an exercise physiologist at Brigham Young University in Utah.

"Also, as you eat less and lose weight, your metabolism slows, and weight loss slows along with it," explains weight-loss expert George Blackburn, M.D., Ph.D. If you want to keep losing fat and maintain muscle mass, your best bet is to step up your walking program.

Finally, pay attention to what you do, not what you lose. "There are some things in life you can't control, and weight is one of them," says Dr. Fischer. "Even if you do everything right, you can't always lose as much weight as you've planned. So if you strive only for weight loss, you'll get discouraged. But you can control behavior that leads to weight loss. Work for goals you can achieve."

Walk for as long as you feel comfortable, even if it seems ridiculously short. "For someone who gets out of breath just going up a flight of stairs, a walk to the end of the driveway and back is a big deal," says Gail Johnston, the director of the Aerobics and Fitness Association of America's specialty certification program, Fitness for the Overweight. "Give yourself credit for whatever you can do—don't blame yourself for what you can't."

So let your breathing be your guide. If a daily 5-minute walk is the most you can bear, then so be it. And when you become comfortable with that much, increase it by another 5 minutes. The point is to walk a little every day. Just be patient. You'll see results in good time. After all, the more slowly you lose your weight, the more likely it will stay lost.

HURDLE #4:
YOU DON'T FEEL LIKE THE
SAME PERSON

As you lose more and more weight, you'll start to look like a new person. And people may treat you differently. Some people have difficulty adjusting to their new role. "One of my clients used fat as an excuse to hibernate and not go out with men," says psychologist Susan Olson, Ph.D. "When she lost weight and started dating, she felt like she was dealing with 28-year-old men at a 14-year-old's level. She hadn't built social skills."

You may get negative reactions from friends and lovers, generally the result of jealousy.

The key solution is to confront the problems—not panic and regain the weight, says psychologist Barbara Jacobson, Ph.D. It may seem easier to live with your familiar fat problems, but you can cope with the new challenges. Discuss your concerns with your spouse or friends. Join a support group if you like. And if your friends reject the new you, it may be a good riddance. "In our opinion, any relationship that is dependent on one partner's obesity and lack of self-esteem is not worth saving," says Dr. Jacobson.

Maintaining the Loss

This plan—which calls for a moderate reduction in fat calories combined with a gradual increase in caloric expenditure through easy exercise—should melt away about 1 to 2 pounds per week. That's exactly the rate that experts say brings a steady, permanent weight loss.

To maintain the loss, then, you may be able to eat a little more than while you were losing but less than what you ate before making the commitment to a lower weight. "Keep in mind that for every pound you lose, you will burn 10 calories less per day just because you are lighter," says Dr. Blackburn.

"So, to maintain a 30-pound loss, you'll have to eat 300 calories a day less or burn 300 calories a day more than you did at your higher weight."

The good news is that if you've succeeded at taking off 30-plus pounds, you've already adopted the kind of positive habits you'll need to maintain the loss for life.

Put One Foot in Front of the Other— And Leave the Pounds Behind

Walking is a great way to lose weight. Many weight-loss experts are now mapping out special programs for people who want to lose.

But sometimes having the right map isn't enough to get you out on the road. You need a little coaching, a little encouragement in the day-to-day effort.

Joe Owens, professor of exercise physiology and director of the fitness laboratory at the State University of New York at New Paltz, has been in the fitness business for 34 years. A former coach, athletic director and consultant, he's stacked up plenty of tips for staying motivated. Here are some encouraging words from the coach.

Have a Specific Goal • Create goals that allow you to achieve a little bit every day or every week. Too often people create unmanageable goals, like "I want to be a millionaire," and they never feel the satisfaction of reaching a less dramatic goal.

Plan to walk a certain amount every day, based on your ability. Each day you achieve your goal, give yourself a mental pat on the back. If you miss a day, don't punish yourself. Give yourself encouragement even when you walk less than your goal.

Visualize Your Goal • Being able to see, feel, hear, and taste your goal is a powerful force in reaching it. Olympians imagine the roar of the crowds, the applause, the feeling of the gold medal being placed around their neck. They use all their senses to visualize their goal to keep motivation high.

You can do the same thing. Feel what it would be like to be walking at a brisk pace on a cool morning. Imagine what you'll feel like when you've achieved your weight-loss goal and you're still out there walking to maintain it. Imagine how much healthier you'll feel, how much easier your body will move, how the strength in your muscles will power you along, how much easier your breathing will be. Feel the new energy your walking program will bring you.

Find a Role Model • Find a person you'd like to emulate, a person who walks regularly and maintains her weight. What are her strategies for getting out there every day and walking? Copy them! Identifying with a positive role model can be a real shortcut to success.

Take Steps to Improve Your Mental Attitude • Take steps, literally! If you want to improve your mental attitude toward walking, get out and walk. Some experts feel that walking improves your sense of well-being. Tell yourself you have a goal but that you're going to enjoy the battle even more than the victory. Get that mind/body loop going!

Make a List and Check It Twice • Make a list of as many reasons as you can brainstorm for why you want to maintain a regular walking program. You can't think of too many things!

"I can wear designer jeans. I'll perform better. I'll sleep better, eat better, get off some medication, eat more of the things that I like, feel more psychologically balanced, do better at work." Keep going!

Then make a list of the reasons that you can't get out and walk regularly. You want to know something? That list will be a lot harder to compile!

Then match those lists. The good things you achieve will far outnumber the reasons for not doing the walking. Owens

THREE WAYS TO STEP UP YOUR WEIGHT-LOSS PROGRAM

Walking at any speed will burn calories, but if you want to increase the calorie-burn potential of your daily walking workout, you can:

1. Walk farther. Every extra mile can smoke off another 100 calories. If you're pressed for time, gradually get accustomed to walking a little faster.

2. Add a few hills to your workout. Even a slight incline can increase your effort and eat up calories!

3. Wear a weight belt or weighted vest. Hand weights may alter your stride or cause you to injure your arms or shoulders.

says he likes to challenge people who want to lose weight to give him ten reasons that they can't, without repeating themselves. They can't do it!

Tips to Lose By

By George L. Blackburn, M.D., Ph.D.

In our weight-loss programs at the New England Deaconess Hospital in Boston, we've supervised thousands of successful diets. Following are some of the tips and techniques our staff has found work best.

Get in Control

First, here are some tricks to quash your appetite.

Eat Your Breakfast • Mom was right: You shouldn't skip meals, especially not breakfast. Breakfast serves as a "metabolic kicker." The body needs fluids and a range of nutrients in the morning to get started. And breakfast will ward off the afternoon munchies. If you really can't stomach food in the morning, a good-quality instant breakfast product is a better solution than nothing. (Look for a product that's low in sugar and that provides a third of the nutrient Recommended Dietary Allowances.)

Steer Clear of Sweets • Don't eat sugary breakfasts (or snacks). Sugar stimulates the appetite. It also gives you a quick boost of energy, which is often followed by a depressing fall.

Eat a Variety of Foods • A good meal should include three types of food—three different colors—at several different temperatures. This kind of eating is best for your body and triggers feelings of satisfaction.

Slow Down • When you do eat, take your time. A meal should last at least 20 or, ideally, 30 minutes. You need time to chew thoroughly, to concentrate on enjoying the sensations of eating: taste and smell. You'll feel more satisfied.

Try the Carb Trick • Start your meal with a high-carbohydrate food, like a pasta appetizer, bread without butter, or a bean or noodle soup. That should lessen your fat craving as the meal wears on, and then you won't be as likely to want a high-fat dessert.

Get Moving

One of the best ways to lose weight is to step up your activity level.

Burn Your Fat • I believe the effectiveness of exercise in burning fat depends not on how hard you move, but how steadily. If someone wants to weigh about 10 percent less, they're going to have to move their bodies an average of 200 minutes a week, and many people will have to move 400 minutes a week. What do those minutes of movement do? They encourage the fat to leave the adipose tissue, where it is stored, to go into the bloodstream and then the liver, where it is burned. If you're not active, any fat you lose by dieting will simply recirculate in the blood and return to the adipose tissue.

Watch the Clock • Contrary to popular belief, you don't have to shed a lot of sweat, blood, and tears to lose weight! You just have to move your body on a sustained basis—ideally 15 minutes at a time—for a total of 30 minutes to an hour a day, or 200 to 400 minutes each week. That activity can be anything from vacuuming and making beds to climbing stairs or walking.

Get Motivated

Changing fattening behavior patterns is another effective strategy. Here are some suggestions.

Set Small Goals • Set small, realistic goals each week. Not weight-loss goals; behavior goals. Example: You know lunch is a problem for you because you're always tempted by cafeteria desserts. Your first week's goal is to pack along a healthy lunch on two workdays. Next week, make it three days, and so on.

Write It Down • Keep a food diary, which includes not only what you eat, but when and where. You'll be able to identify patterns and "food cues" (like the cafeteria desserts) that stimulate you to overeat.

Get Smart

And finally, keep these keys to a healthy diet in mind as you pursue your weight-loss goals.

Limit Your Fat • Learning to limit fat intake is the most important step you can take, for health as well as weight loss. Our clients are given a book that lists grams of fat in common foods, and they learn how to keep fat consumption beneath 30 percent of their ideal daily calorie intake. (That's about 40 to 50 grams of fat each day for the average woman, and 60 to 70 grams for the average man.) A nutritionist can help you calculate the limits that are appropriate for you.

Learn Ten New Recipes • Most people have about ten recipes that they enjoy and use again and again. If you can learn ten alternative, low-fat recipes that you enjoy cooking and eating, you'll go a long way toward ensuring a healthy diet.

Know When to Stop • Our clients go on a maintenance diet after 12 weeks of low-calorie eating. They maintain their weight for at least three to six months. Then, if they need to, they can start weight loss again. This avoids burnout and means their set point—the weight their metabolism wants to maintain—is readjusted gradually, making the change more likely to stick.

The Diet for Diehard Snackers

Thus sayeth the nutritional Law of the Land: Eat just three meals a day and no between-meal snacks. But a whole lot of people have been breaking this commandment since day one. They're nibblers, or grazers—eating four, five, six mini-meals or snacks throughout the day. And surprisingly enough, some nutritional research suggests that the nibbling habit, if carefully monitored, may actually be a good way for some people to control weight—which is especially welcome news to dieters, because they're already prone to nibbling. They're actually more likely to snack than nondieters, one survey shows.

One of nibbling's advantages in weight control is that it can lead to more calorie burning than the usual three-meals-a-day scheme. "If you consume about 1,500 calories between 6:00 and 9:00 P.M.—which you could easily do by eating a conventional dinner—that food won't be fully digested and ready for use until 2:00 A.M.," says Helen A. Guthrie, Ph.D., professor of nutrition at Pennsylvania State University. "By then, you're not burning many calories because you're asleep. So your body stores most of the calories as fat. If you don't eat breakfast, your body will draw on some of that fat for energy—but not all of it."

But by judicious nibbling, you avoid piling up most of your daily calories in the evening—you spread them out over the entire day in six or more little meals. You consume most of your calories when you're active, when your calorie burning is in overdrive. And if you reserve part of your day for exercise (an essential part of any weight-control plan), you can help the whole process along. Even a 20- to 30-minute daily walk can substantially crank up your body's calorie-burn rate.

Another point for nibbling: It may increase the body's absorption of vitamins and minerals, which can be a big advantage over many weight-loss plans that call for eating less food and therefore getting fewer essential nutrients. Let's say two diets are exactly equal in vitamin and mineral content. The only difference: One consists of one or two big meals, while the other consists of several smaller meals. "The body will absorb a higher percentage of most nutrients from a series of smaller meals than it will from one or two large meals," says John Pinto, Ph.D., director of the nutrition research laboratory at Memorial Sloan-Kettering Hospital. "So the total amount of nutrients absorbed from the smaller meals will be higher."

Which is not to say that a nibble weight-loss plan would work for everyone. "In people who have trouble stopping eating once they begin, exposure to food six times a day may double the temptation to overeat," says Kelly Brownell, Ph.D., a weight-loss specialist and psychologist at the University of Pennsylvania School of Medicine.

On the other hand, some diehard snackers may find a nibble diet the easiest in the world to stick to. It may help stifle the temptation to overindulge by offering something to eat every 2 to 3 hours.

With all this in mind, this nibble diet is tailor-made for all those who've dreamed of losing weight while eating far more than three squares a day.

How It Works

This six-meals-a-day diet consists of breakfast, lunch, and dinner plus three planned snacks, with plenty of variety built in for fun. Total daily calorie intake, of course, is reduced to ensure gradual weight loss. And the proportion of calories in each meal is calibrated for maximum enjoyment and fat fighting.

For each of the six mealtimes, the accompanying lists give you ideas for at least seven planned menus—enough tantalizing mealtime options to keep you nibbling for days without enjoying the same meal twice. And all the suggested menus feature the Three Essential Elements of Lose-Weight Nibbling:

1. The meals are low in fat, because dietary fat is more easily converted into body fat than either carbohydrates or protein.

2. They can be whipped together in a flash—generally in 30 minutes or less; many in 5 or 10 minutes flat. After all, nibbling almost always calls for fast food.

3. The menus are designed for optimum variety and taste (because even nibbling can get boring if you're not careful).

Not only are all 49 menus different, but you can add all the "no-limit" foods to them you want (check the list of these foods in "Freebies"). You can eat each meal whenever you want (letting hunger be your guide). And you can do some substituting from one mealtime to another. Breakfast and lunch menus can be switched, for example, and so can menus for the midmorning and midafternoon snacks. (Snacks shouldn't be traded for "main meals," though, and dinners and evening snacks shouldn't be traded at all.) Plus, you can alter any menu, as long as you keep the amount of fat and calories about the same.

FREEBIES

You may add the following items to any meal or snack at any time: celery; lettuce; parsley sprigs; radishes; coffee (with artificial sweetener); herbal tea (with artificial sweetener); seltzer, any amount; tea (with artificial sweetener); water, any amount; "lite" ketchup; mustard; oil-free Italian salad dressing; salsa; soy sauce; steak sauce; Tabasco sauce; white-wine Worcestershire sauce; Worcestershire sauce; any spices, no limit; sugar-free gelatin.

The Nibbler's Weight-Loss Plan

The version of our nibble diet presented here is based on an intake of 1,500 calories a day. Adjust calorie levels up or down if weight loss is slower or faster than the 1 to 2 pounds per week recommended by doctors. To adjust for a higher caloric intake, increase the portion sizes of the lower-fat foods. Piling on more of the higher-fat items could add pounds as well as calories.

Breakfast

1. Two slices french toast, made with two egg whites, one yolk, and minced mandarin orange (canned); one fresh peach or one half, canned in juice.

2. One serving bran-type cereal with skim milk; grapefruit half; 8 ounces tomato juice; one slice white or whole wheat toast with 1 teaspoon all-fruit spread.

3. Three buckwheat pancakes, 4-inch diameter, made with skim milk; "lite" syrup; one orange.

4. Instant oatmeal with added raisins and cinnamon; one banana; two pieces melba toast with light coating of margarine.

5. One bagel with 1 teaspoon all-fruit spread; 6 ounces orange juice.

6. One large biscuit shredded wheat cereal with $\frac{1}{2}$ cup skim milk; one banana; one slice white or whole wheat toast with 1 teaspoon all-fruit spread.

7. Two waffles with 2 tablespoons "lite" syrup; one fresh tangerine, or $\frac{1}{3}$ cup canned tangerines in light syrup.

Midmorning Snack

1. One banana; five vanilla wafers.

2. One slice raisin bread with 1 teaspoon all-fruit spread; one fresh pear, or two halves, canned in juice.

3. Eight ounces plain yogurt with either one-half banana, $\frac{1}{2}$ cup blueberries, 10 cherries, $\frac{1}{2}$ cup orange slices, $\frac{1}{2}$ cup peach slices, $\frac{3}{4}$ cup raspberries, 1 cup strawberries, or one tangerine.

4. One grapefruit (peel and eat it like an orange!); one-half toasted English muffin with light coating of margarine or all-fruit spread.

5. Twelve ounces orange juice or grapefruit juice; one rice cake with 1 tablespoon all-fruit spread.

6. Three applesauce muffins (see recipe on page 118) with light coating of margarine.

7. Five wafers melba toast or Norwegian crispbread with 1 tablespoon homemade sweet yogurt cheese (see recipe on page 117) on each wafer.

8. Twelve ounces skim or low-fat milk; three squares graham cracker.

Lunch

1. Pita pocket sandwich with tuna fish, lettuce, and tomato slices; two gingersnaps.

2. Large salad with 3 to 4 tablespoons creamy dressing (see recipe on page 116); ½ cup pinto or navy beans, cooked and chilled, served in spiced vinegar or over the salad; one orange.

3. Four slices lean roast beef on whole wheat bread, with lettuce and mustard; one raw carrot; one banana.

4. Cold pasta salad with light vinaigrette (or oil-free Italian dressing); one tangerine.

5. Pita pocket with chicken, tomato, and lettuce; three stalks celery; two plums or two large prunes.

6. One and one-half cups three-bean salad made with kidney beans, green beans, and wax beans; one raw carrot; one Bartlett or d'Anjou pear.

7. Eight ounces plain yogurt with either one-half banana, ½ cup blueberries, 10 cherries, ½ cup orange slices, ½ cup peach slices, ¾ cup raspberries, 1 cup strawberries, or one tangerine; three gingersnaps.

8. Three deli slices turkey breast on whole wheat bread, with lettuce and 1 tablespoon all-fruit spread; one peach.

Midafternoon Snack

1. Three fig bars.

2. Eight or nine thin pretzels.

3. Apple; 1½ graham crackers.

4. Six wafers melba toast or Norwegian crispbread with 1 tablespoon homemade savory yogurt cheese (see recipe on page 117) on each wafer.

5. Three cups air-popped popcorn; 8 ounces canned apple juice.

6. Five wafers melba toast or Norwegian crispbread with 1 tablespoon homemade hummus (see recipe on page 118) on each wafer.

7. One peach; three rice cakes with 1 tablespoon all-fruit spread on each.

Dinner

1. Six ounces broiled or baked salmon; $\frac{3}{4}$ cup frozen or canned peas; 1 cup fresh or frozen cauliflower; small salad with 1 to 2 tablespoons creamy dressing (see recipe on page 116).

2. One-half baked or broiled chicken breast; baked potato; 1 cup red cabbage with apple slices; medium salad with 2 tablespoons creamy dressing (see recipe on page 116).

3. Eight ocean (large) scallops or 20 bay (small) scallops, baked or broiled; 1 cup mashed potatoes made with skim milk; 2 spears fresh broccoli or 1 cup chopped frozen broccoli; medium salad with 2 tablespoons creamy dressing (see recipe on page 116).

4. Five ounces broiled sirloin steak (trimmed of all fat before cooking); one pepper and one large onion, sliced and broiled with steak; 1 cup canned or frozen string beans; small salad with 1 to 2 tablespoons creamy dressing (see recipe on page 116).

5. Three slices turkey breast; $\frac{3}{4}$ cup brown or white rice; one raw carrot or $\frac{2}{3}$ cup cooked carrots; small salad with 1 to 2 tablespoons creamy dressing (see recipe on page 116).

6. Seven ounces baked or broiled flounder; one ear corn, 7 to 8 inches long, or $\frac{3}{4}$ cup frozen or canned corn; 1 cup cooked fresh or frozen spinach; medium salad with 2 tablespoons creamy dressing (see recipe on page 116).

7. One baked or broiled chicken leg, drumstick and thigh, with skin removed; one baked sweet potato; two raw green or red peppers; medium salad with 2 tablespoons creamy dressing (see recipe on page 116).

8. One frozen chicken enchilada (add salsa to taste); $\frac{1}{2}$ cup canned refried beans; small salad with lettuce, tomato, sweet and hot peppers.

9. One and one-half cups spaghetti (or any other pasta) with ¾ cup meatless tomato sauce, spiced to taste; medium salad with 2 tablespoon creamy dressing (see recipe below) or "lite" Italian dressing.

Evening Snack
    1. Three cups air-popped popcorn.
    2. One and one-half scoops sherbet, any flavor.
    3. One small slice angel food cake.
    4. One-half cup applesauce; two gingersnaps.
    5. One-half cup sugar-free pudding, any flavor, made with skim or 2 percent milk.
    6. One-half cantaloupe.
    7. About 30 seedless grapes.
    8. One scoop ice milk.
    9. Ten dried apricots.
    10. Three slices pineapple, canned in juice.

Recipes for the Nibbler

Cool, Creamy Dressing

1 cup nonfat cottage cheese

¼ cup skim milk

1 tablespoon lemon juice

½ teaspoon Dijon-style mustard

1 clove garlic, minced

1 tablespoon minced parsley

1 tablespoon minced fresh basil or ½ teaspoon dried basil

In a blender or food processor, puree the cottage cheese, milk, lemon juice, mustard, and garlic until smooth. Transfer to a medium bowl. Stir in the parsley and basil (another herb may be used for variety). If too thick, thin with skim milk or nonfat yogurt.

Makes about 1 cup (average serving size: 2 tablespoons; 20 calories per serving)

Sweet or Savory Yogurt Cheese

Basic Yogurt Cheese

3 cups plain nonfat yogurt

Line a colander with cheesecloth and spoon in yogurt. Let drain in the refrigerator overnight.
Makes about 1½ cups (15 calories per tablespoon)

Orange Almond Cheese

1½ cups yogurt cheese

 2 tablespoons minced raisins

 1 tablespoon chopped almonds

1½ teaspoons honey

1½ teaspoons orange juice concentrate, thawed

 ⅛ teaspoon ground cinnamon

Combine ingredients in a medium bowl.
Makes about 1½ cups (22 calories per tablespoon)

Herbal Yogurt Cheese

1½ cups yogurt cheese

 1 clove garlic, minced

 1 tablespoon minced parsley

 1 teaspoon dried herbs (try combinations such as
    dill/savory, tarragon/chervil, rosemary/thyme, and
    others)

Combine ingredients in a medium bowl.
Makes about 1½ cups (16 calories per tablespoon)

Hummus

1½ cups canned chick-peas

¼ cup water

3 tablespoons lemon juice

1 tablespoon tahini (sesame-seed paste)

1 teaspoon olive oil

¾ teaspoon garlic powder

½ teaspoon ground cumin

   Pinch of ground red pepper

½ cup chopped coriander leaves

In a blender or food processor, puree the chick-peas, water, lemon juice, tahini, oil, garlic powder, cumin, and pepper until smooth. Transfer to a medium bowl and stir in coriander.

Makes 1½ cups (24 calories per tablespoon)

Applesauce Muffins

1 cup oat bran

⅓ cup whole wheat flour

½ cup bran

2 teaspoons baking powder

⅓ teaspoon ground cinnamon

2 egg whites

⅓ cup applesauce

1 cup skim milk

½ cup blueberries, raspberries, chopped peaches, mashed
     bananas, or shredded apples

Coat a 12-cup muffin tin with vegetable cooking spray.

   In a large bowl, combine the oat bran, flour, bran, baking powder, and cinnamon. Set aside.

   Preheat oven to 425°F.

   In a medium bowl, combine the egg whites and applesauce. Whisk in the skim milk, then pour liquid into flour mixture. Mix until moistened. Fold in the fruit. Spoon batter into prepared muffin tin and bake 15 to 18 minutes, or until muffins are lightly browned.

Makes 12 muffins (about 60 calories each)

Curb Your Cravings for Fat

By George L. Blackburn, M.D., Ph.D.

Got a hankering for fat? Few of us would admit that we do. But cravings for ice cream, chocolate bars, french fries, or juicy T-bones are, for the most part, fat cravings.

Everyone has a "fat tooth," although some people crave fat more than others. That's because each of us is programmed to crave foods with a taste, texture, and sensation that reflect a certain ratio of fat to carbohydrate. In other words, it's this personal fat-to-carbohydrate ratio that determines what we think are the best-tasting foods. And that ratio differs from person to person. It's dictated by genetics and environmental factors, including ethnic background. Researchers have observed this ratio in operation in young children. When presented with a smorgasbord, fourth-graders' selections were quite different (in fat-to-carbohydrate ratio) from one another. But, on consecutive days, each child chose foods with a fat-to-carbohydrate ratio that was consistent with his or her own selections the day before.

The problem with this fat craving is that most nutritionists consider fat to be the number-one diet enemy of good health.

First, fat makes you fat. High-fat foods are richer in calories. And calories from fat "count more" than calories from carbohydrates. The fats you eat are easily stored as fat, whereas carbohydrates have to be converted to fat—a process that burns calories. This effect is so significant that studies show that people who start to replace some of their calories from fat with some from carbohydrates shed an average of 5 pounds in four to six weeks. Without their old high-fat, favorite-foods diet, they ate less and burned more body fat and calories.

If you're overweight, losing those extra pounds can have a profound effect on your health. Excess body weight contributes to diabetes, high blood pressure, and heart disease.

A high-fat diet also encourages heart disease by helping along the artery-clogging process. And it's believed to increase the risk of developing certain forms of cancer.

There is even some evidence that fat contributes to immune-related disorders, including viral and bacterial infections. Fats are precursors of prostaglandins, substances that regulate our immune system. There's some indication that more fat in the diet can influence prostaglandins in a way that weakens our immune system.

Breaking Free of Fat

Unfortunately, most Americans eat too much fat—about 40 percent of total calories. That amounts to about 71 to 107 grams of fat a day for the average woman and about 102 to 138 grams for the average man. To maintain proper weight and good health, your best bet is to limit the number of fat calories you eat to less than 30 percent of total intake. Target fat intake should be between 53 and 80 grams a day for women and less than 103 grams for men. A dietitian can help you estimate the fat in your current diet.

(Some Pritikin-type approaches suggest you decrease fat consumption even more—to 20 percent of your calories. This may be sensible for some people, particularly those who have plaque formation in their arteries. You can discuss this with your doctor or dietitian.) Keep in mind that the central health issue is: How much total fat are you eating? At this stage, it really doesn't matter whether you're eating butter or margarine, saturated animal fat or monounsaturated olive oil. Fat is fat. You've got to cut it across the board.

In Southeast Asia, for example, the predominant fat the people consume is coconut oil, which is about 90 percent saturated. Yet they have the lowest incidence of heart disease in the world, and the lowest cholesterol levels, because their total fat intake is low.

In fact, research shows that 75 percent of people see health benefits when they move from a high-fat to a low-fat diet. After total fat intake is reduced, another 6 percent of people benefit from replacing saturated fats with a balance of polyunsaturated and monounsaturated fats (found in vegetable, fish, and olive and canola oils).

Tricking Your Fat Tooth

Of course, it's not so easy to reduce your fat consumption. Your fat-to-carbohydrate ratio creates cravings that are hard to resist.

There is one trick you can use to diminish the power of your fat tooth, though. It's called "carbohydrate preloading." Here's how it works.

The first thing you eat at a meal should be a starch or carbohydrate. Soups that contain noodles, potatoes, rice, barley, or legumes are excellent choices. Try mushroom, barley, pasta e fagioli, or split-pea soup. Or start with a small serving of spaghetti with tomato sauce. Low-fat whole wheat bread is another perfect food for preloading. (No croissants!) If you're at a restaurant, French bread can do the trick—just skip the butter. Then try to "stretch out" the meal. Eat slowly and take time between courses so it lasts for at least 20 minutes. That gives the carbohydrates time to activate the hormones in your intestinal tract, liver, and brain, so you won't feel as much of a craving for fat as you go on with the meal. (Of course, planning meals with less fat, including low-fat desserts, is important, too. Try angel-food cake with strawberries to satisfy your desire for something sweet without raising your fat intake.)

You can apply this principle when you get snack cravings, too. Often, what people think is a sweet craving is actually a fat craving. Treats like ice cream and candy bars are high in sugar, but they're also high in fat. So plan snacks that are low in fat and high in carbohydrates. When you do get that 4 o'clock yearning, have a glass of skim milk with an apple, for example. The high-carbohydrate apple can help you ward off fat cravings for several hours.

If you rely on carbohydrate preloading, you may be surprised to find that you can actually eat more food than before. But you'll be eating less fat, and that's your goal.

Super-Nutrient Frontiers

Why You May Need More Iron

No blood. That's what "anemia" literally means. A bit of an exaggeration—but at times it feels true to those who suffer from it. They're tired, light-headed. In severe cases, their pulse rate goes up, blood pressure goes down, and they feel dizzy and weak.

The problem? Their blood lacks enough oxygen-carrying red cells. As a result, every tissue and organ becomes starved for oxygen. Anemics are slowly smothering—from within. The most common cause: not enough iron. Without sufficient iron, the body can't manufacture enough new red blood cells packed with hemoglobin, the red-cell protein that transports the oxygen.

Even mild anemia is an advanced symptom of iron deficiency, since the body will deplete its store of iron before cutting back on blood formation. Looked at another way, it's possible to be iron deficient without being anemic.

One cause of iron-deficiency anemia is blood loss. Women's iron reserves—lower than men's to begin with—can be strained to the limit by menstruation. Men are rarely anemic, but when they are, the cause is usually an ulcer or hemorrhoids.

The Diet Factor

But another big factor in this kind of anemia—which doctors see in mild forms all the time—is diet. This sounds odd, because in this country iron-rich and iron-fortified foods are abundant, and people seem to be more conscious of healthy eating habits than ever.

But strangely enough, the very dietary habits that are bona fide heart healthy can set you up for iron deficiency if you're not careful.

Here's how: Let's say you eat a breakfast of two large biscuits of shredded wheat with ½ cup of skim milk, one slice of whole wheat toast and one cup of coffee. You lunch on a fresh garden salad, ½ cup of cottage cheese, iced tea, and 1 cup of grapes. Then in the evening you dine on 4 ounces of broiled bluefish, ½ cup of boiled, fresh carrots, 1 cup of long-grain rice, a cup of tea with honey and lemon and one slice of apple pie. And for a late-night snack, you polish off a cup of yogurt with a fresh peach.

What could possibly be wrong with this diet? It's low in fat and cholesterol, high in fiber—it even has calcium. But it might put you on the wrong side of the iron curtain.

First, it's sorely lacking in iron—only 6.73 milligrams, a far cry from the Recommended Dietary Allowance (RDA) of 18 milligrams for women 50 and younger and 10 milligrams for women over 50 and men. The main reason is that iron-rich foods like red meat have been omitted to reduce intake of fat and cholesterol. Second, the combination of foods may be a problem. Components of the foods may interact with dietary iron to actually decrease the amount of iron the body absorbs.

The good news is that it's possible to avoid these roads to iron deficiency without switching to the liver 'n' onions blue plate special. Here are some simple ways to modify a diet like the one above to keep it heart healthy and iron strong.

Choose Lean Meats • The iron in meat isn't hiding in the fat. So, moderate-sized portions of lean red meat will give you lots of iron without sabotaging your low-fat regimen. Chicken and some fish (generally lower in saturated fat than red meat) are also good sources of iron.

And not only does meat contain iron, it has the kind of iron most useful to your body. "Dietary iron occurs in two forms, heme and nonheme," says Marvin Adner, M.D., director of hematology at Framingham Union Hospital in Massachusetts. "Very simply, heme iron is the type that forms hemoglobin; it comes only from animal sources and it's readily absorbed by the body. Nonheme iron is any other form of iron; it's found in plants, but it's not as easily absorbed."

Eat Vegetables and Grains with Lean Meat • "Popeye lied— spinach is not a great source of iron. One study found that only 1.5 percent of its nonheme iron is absorbed," says Victor Herbert, M.D., professor of medicine at Mount Sinai and Bronx Veterans Administration Medical Centers. In fact, the average percentage of iron that can be absorbed from most plant sources alone is 3 percent. But eating meat with spinach or any other nonheme iron source can boost that figure.

The reason is that some as-yet-unidentified substance called "animal protein factor" enhances the absorption of plant iron when meat and vegetables are eaten together. This animal protein factor is found only in meat, poultry, and fish.

Beware the Calcium Effect • Milk and cheese don't contain animal protein factor. In fact, they can slightly inhibit iron absorption, primarily because of a high calcium and phosphate content. That doesn't mean cut back on calcium, but it would be wise not to combine an iron-rich meal with too many cheese sauces and milk shakes. Neither is it a good idea to take iron supplements and calcium supplements together, since the calcium will bind with the iron. If you must take both, take them at different times of the day.

Eat Iron-Rich Legumes • Dried beans and peas are the most iron-rich plant products in our diet. True, the legumes' non-heme iron isn't as well absorbed as iron from meat. But many other plant sources don't have much iron at all. Three percent absorption of 4.5 milligrams of iron in a cup of dried beans, for example, is better than 3 percent of the 0.3 milligrams in iceberg lettuce. And if you eat some meat along with beans, you can bump that 3 percent way up.

Combine Iron-Rich Foods with Foods High in Vitamin C • More good news for vegetarians: Vitamin C enhances the absorption of nonheme iron in vegetables, fruits, and fortified cereals. A glass of orange juice with breakfast can more than double the amount of iron your body absorbs. Some studies have found that vitamin C can increase overall iron absorption threefold to sixfold. The trick is to make sure you eat the vitamin C foods with the iron foods. They work only when eaten together.

Get Your Fiber, But . . . • Here's another piece of dual-edged data: Dietary fiber may help lower cholesterol, yet too much fiber inhibits nonheme iron absorption. It's because some types of fiber like bran bind to nonheme iron and move through the digestive system quickly, giving the iron little chance to be absorbed. This might spell trouble for someone with a low-iron, high-fiber diet. The answer? Don't cut down on fiber, just don't overdo it. As long as your daily fiber intake doesn't exceed about 30 grams, you needn't worry—especially if you follow the tips given here.

Avoid Drinking Tea or Coffee with Your Meals • And don't wash down an iron supplement with a mug of java. The tannins in these beverages bind with iron, making less of it available. A cup of tea with breakfast can block three-fourths of the iron that you would have absorbed.

Cook Foods in an Iron Pot Whenever Practical • In our grand-mothers' time, the iron that leached into food from iron pots and pans acted as a kind of unintentional fortification. In one study, spaghetti sauce simmered in an iron pot for about 20 minutes increased its iron content ninefold. Granted, the pot can only add nonheme iron, but it can make a big difference in your diet.

Eat Iron-Fortified Foods • Iron-fortified or enriched breakfast cereals and other foods can help boost your iron intake. But you shouldn't rely on them exclusively, because the iron in them isn't always very absorbable.

Three types of nonheme iron are used to fortify foods: ferrous compounds, ferric compounds, and electrolytic iron. Ferrous compounds, such as ferrous sulfate, are well absorbed. The problem is that they're highly reactive—in storage they can change the color, odor, and taste of some foods. When manufacturers found that their cereal smelled like rotten fish, they switched to less reactive and less well absorbed ferric compounds (beginning with "ferric," like ferric pyrophosphate).

The nonreactive yet well-absorbed alternative is electrolytic iron, also known as elemental iron or "reduced iron." If a food is fortified with vitamin C as well, quite a bit of the iron will be absorbed.

So when food labels spell out what kind of iron is used, go for the more absorbable types. When labels simply state "iron" without any qualification (which is how they're usually labeled), remember that some of the iron will get absorbed no matter what kind it is. And then there's always o.j. and other C-packed foods to help the absorption process along.

Consider Supplements • If you're a young woman (especially if you're dieting), you should evaluate your diet and decide if you need iron supplements. Many doctors say that if you're pregnant, you should be taking supplements, since it's extremely difficult to meet your increased RDA (30 to 60 milligrams) at the dinner table. Most other people except anemics, experts say, probably don't need supplements. (A hint: If you take supplements, do it at night, on an empty stomach, along with some orange juice. This helps ensure minimum stomach upset and maximum absorption.)

The down-sides of iron supplements are few. Some people experience stomach irritation from them. In a rare hereditary condition called hemochromatosis, supplements can cause serious iron overloading.

If you have an iron deficiency, your doctor may recommend either iron supplements or iron-fortified foods or both.

On the Verge of Cancer Breakthroughs

First, scientists analyzed the protective effect of fiber. Then they studied the ill effects of fat. Now, they're picking up where theories left off to determine what other food factors can give us the edge against cancer. Five essential nutrients have taken the lead. Coming right up—a review of the evidence.

Vitamin A

Vitamin A, in the form of retin-A ointment, has made the headlines recently as a wrinkle reducer. But other forms and relatives of this vitamin—especially beta-carotene—have been winning special attention for their potential role in reducing cancer. Back in the 1920s, a researcher reported that a diet deficient in vitamin A appeared to cause stomach cancer in rats.

A follow-up study showed that the rats had actually developed a precancerous condition, not a full-fledged cancer. But, in cancer research, that is considered significant. And the vitamin A/cancer connection was established.

Since then, scientists have demonstrated that, in animals, vitamin A inhibits precancerous changes—and in some cases, cancer—in the prostate, bladder, and breast. And the findings aren't just "mildly intriguing." One study showed that a synthetic vitamin-A compound blocked one-fifth of the expected breast tumors in animals pretreated with a potent cancer-causing chemical.

Turning to human populations, researchers have logged additional evidence. In Norway, male smokers were asked to keep a food diary, then were ranked according to their vitamin A index. Those whose diets ranked low in the vitamin had a higher lung cancer risk. In Japan, a ten-year study involving over 250,000 people (7,377 of whom developed cancer) found a similar link. Daily diets high in beta-carotene were associated with decreased risks of cancers of the lung, colon, stomach, prostate, and cervix. In study after study, there appears to be evidence that diets high in vitamin A and beta-carotene offer protection against certain types of cancer—especially cancers involving the lining of the lungs, throat, stomach, colon, and cervix (the epithelial tissues).

Granted, this evidence is considered preliminary. None of the studies to date has demonstrated a clear cause-and-effect relationship. And, while most have pointed to vitamin A's potential protective effect, there are some inconsistencies in the research. Some studies failed to show that vitamin A had any effect at all on certain precancerous conditions. Others suggest that it may have a negative effect in the prostate. Then, of course, there's the problem that vitamin A, a fat-soluble nutrient, is toxic in high doses.

Current Research • Scientists have now turned the spotlight on beta-carotene, a water-soluble compound that's converted to vitamin A in the body. Beta-carotene is abundant in carrots, green and orange vegetables, and other plants (as opposed to vitamin A, which is found exclusively in meat—especially liver—eggs, and milk). Unlike vitamin A, excesses of beta-carotene are not stored in the liver where they can do damage.

Beta-carotene's safety record and cancer-preventive potential are so strong that doctors are now volunteering as guinea pigs for the next set of trials. In Boston, 22,000 healthy male physicians—with no known risk of cancer—are leading the way. Every other day, they take a pill—either beta-carotene or a red-colored sugar pill (placebo). When the study ends in 1991, the beta-carotene group will have taken supplements for about seven years—and scientists will know more about beta-carotene's impact on all kinds of cancers. "We're interested in total cancer incidence," says researcher Kim Eberlein, of Brigham and Women's Hospital and Harvard Medical School.

Beta-carotene is the headliner in current lung cancer research, too. Several studies are in progress. In Texas, 630 people are receiving either a combination of beta-carotene and vitamin A or a placebo. All volunteers had been exposed to asbestos, a known cause of cancer. "Studies like mine assume that the protective substance is beta-carotene, but we still don't know," says Jerry McLarty, Ph.D., at the University of Texas Health Center.

Houston researchers have likewise turned their attention to beta-carotene. They've been studying patients with oral leukoplakia, a precancerous condition of the mouth. In a study of 44 patients, they found that 13-cis retinoic acid, a synthetic (and highly toxic) form of vitamin A, reversed precancerous growth in 54 percent of those given the vitamin-A compound (13 patients). Only 10 percent (2 patients) of those given placebos experienced reversal. Now, in a follow-up study, they are testing both 13-cis retinoic acid and beta-carotene. "Many investigators have suggested that beta-carotene is as effective as synthetic vitamin A. And there's no toxicity," says Waun Ki Hong, M.D., a professor of medicine and the principal investigator at M. D. Anderson Cancer Center.

Vitamin C

True or false: If you eat plenty of citrus fruits and vegetables that contain vitamin C, you lower your risk of cancer. Answer: We don't know for sure, but the evidence looks promising. Based on preliminary population studies, vitamin C may have potential in combating precancerous conditions of the colon.

In London, scientists found that vitamin C could slow down the development of colon polyps that are genetically induced (familial polyposis). People with polyps are at greater risk for developing colon cancer.

Current Research • To test the strength of the vitamin C/ polyp link, investigators at New York Hospital have recently completed a study of 60 patients with familial polyposis. One third received vitamins C and E and a high-fiber supplement;

another third the same vitamins with a low-fiber supplement; and the final third received placebos and a low-fiber supplement. "We wanted to block polyp formation," says Jerome J. DeCosse, M.D., Ph.D., of New York Hospital. "I think vitamin C has benefits, but we're waiting for the statisticians to finish their analysis."

Vitamin E

What clued scientists in to the importance of this nutrient? Vitamin E deficiencies in children and farm animals. For 30 years, they've been on the trail of vitamin E, also known as alpha-tocopherol.

In a recent study of over 21,000 Finnish men, researchers found an association between a high blood level of vitamin E and a reduced overall risk of cancer. Other population studies have shown a protective effect for breast cancer and lung cancer. "Lung cancer is one of the areas that looks more promising than others," says William A. Pryor, Ph.D., a professor at Louisiana State University and an expert on vitamin E.

Some researchers believe that, rather than battle cancer by itself, vitamin E may be a "helper" nutrient. It may work with vitamin C, for example, to protect against colon cancer. With selenium, it has been shown to lower the risk of breast cancer in laboratory animals. "Its primary role may be what we call permissive—that is, it's necessary for something else to happen," says Leonard A. Cohen, Ph.D., of the American Health Foundation.

Current Research • In Finland once again, a major vitamin E study is under way. "It's possibly the largest trial involving vitamin E ever carried out," says Hoffman-La Roche scientist Lawrence Machlin, Ph.D., whose company is collaborating with Finnish researchers and the National Cancer Institute. About 26,000 male smokers are receiving a daily dose of either beta-carotene, vitamin E, or a placebo. When the study is completed, in 1993, scientists will be one step closer to understanding the protective effect of these nutrients.

Selenium

Scientists first got interested in selenium because of its toxic effects: Livestock grazing on selenium-laden soil developed corroded hooves. In the course of subsequent research, scientists stumbled on evidence that selenium might reduce the incidence of tumors. That marked the beginning of cancer research with selenium.

In animal experiments, selenium seems to fight hardest against breast and colon cancers. Researchers at the Eppley Institute in Omaha, Nebraska, have found, however, that selenium actually enhanced tumors of the skin and pancreas under some conditions. "This suggests that we can't throw all cancers in together," says Graham Colditz, M.D., a researcher at Harvard Medical School. "We have to stop and look at the relation of selenium to each cancer."

To track the relationship of selenium to cancer in humans, researchers have collected blood samples and followed up to see who developed cancer. So far, a majority of studies have linked higher selenium levels with a lower risk of cancer.

Current Research • In the largest ongoing study of selenium, researchers at the Harvard Medical School are studying a possible link between selenium levels and breast, lung, and colon cancer. The participants, 70,000 women, entered the study by mailing in a set of—are you ready for this?—toenail clippings. "Toenails are a very good indicator of selenium status," says Dr. Colditz, one of the investigators. The first results, analyzing selenium and breast cancer incidence, should be reported soon.

Because the line between "safe" and "dangerous" levels of selenium is small, other researchers are working to develop man-made selenium-containing compounds that have fewer toxic effects but can still suppress tumors. "We are optimistic," says Bandaru S. Reddy, Ph.D., of the American Health Foundation. "Even at higher dose levels, these compounds are not toxic to lab animals and seem to prevent certain cancers very well."

Calcium

Calcium is best known as a barrier to osteoporosis, the weak-bone disease. But cancer researchers suggest it may block cancer, too.

Cedric Garland, Ph.D., and Frank Garland, Ph.D., both of the University of California, San Diego, have detailed a strong, albeit theoretical, link between calcium and cancer. Oddly enough, they took their first clue from some maps of the United States. What they saw was a startling difference in mortality rates for cancer of the breast and intestine between the northern and the Sunbelt states. They speculated that, since sunlight reacts with the skin to create vitamin D, and vitamin D helps the body absorb calcium, perhaps people who live in sunnier climates have healthier calcium levels that protect them against cancer.

To test their theory, they reviewed the dietary questionnaires that 1,954 men had filled out as part of a 20-year study (begun in 1957) on cancer and heart disease. By the time the study had been completed, 49 of the men had developed intestinal cancer.

What the doctors discovered was that those men "ate far fewer foods containing vitamin D and calcium. Men who took in calcium and vitamin D equivalent to 4½ glasses of nonfat milk per day had only about one-third the risk of intestinal cancer."

Other studies suggest that there may be something to this. In Canada, researchers found that people whose diets were supplemented with calcium and vitamin E developed fewer intestinal polyps than a control (nonsupplemented) group. And research at New York's Memorial Sloan-Kettering Cancer Center found that patients who took daily doses of calcium for two to three months slowed the rapid growth of cells lining the large bowel. A high rate of cell division in that portion of the bowel is associated with a high risk of intestinal cancer.

Current Research • Studies involving calcium continue at Memorial Sloan-Kettering Cancer Center. And at M. D. Anderson Cancer Center in Houston, researchers are continuing to study the effects of calcium on colon polyps.

Obviously, the final word isn't in yet—and may not be for a while. In the meantime, take the prudent course, and be sure your intake of these essential nutrients is up to par. (Do keep in mind, too, that taking more than the Recommended Dietary Allowance is not always better; high doses of vitamin A and selenium, for example, can be hazardous to your health.) Your best nutritional hedge against cancer is still a diet that's healthy in every regard: low in fat, high in fiber, and packed with a wide variety of nutrient-dense foods that will meet all your daily requirements—including, of course, vitamins A, C, and E, selenium and calcium.

Boron for Bones

Are your bones getting everything they need to stay healthy and strong?

If not, they could be in big trouble without your even knowing it. Unlike aching joints, which let you know in no uncertain terms when something's not right, the key bones in your legs, hips and spine can shorten, weaken, or break because of osteoporosis with very little advance warning.

We already know a lot about how to prevent this crippling problem. Exercise is one very important factor in the solution, because the more you move, the more your bones are strengthened.

And a diet rich in calcium seems to play a role, too, especially in the younger years, when bone mass is still being built up. Scientists suspect a good head start then could help many women withstand the slow draining away of bone minerals that occurs after menopause.

But research indicates that in some parts of the world, women who get little calcium in their diet still manage somehow to avoid osteoporosis. Could it be that some dietary factor besides calcium is also a vital element in determining bone strength?

A Missing Link?

Scientists at the U.S. Department of Agriculture's (USDA) Human Nutrition Laboratory in Grand Forks, North Dakota, think that might be the case. The substance that's caught their attention is boron, a trace element that's always been in the soil and in our food but often in widely varying amounts. Scientists have long thought that people didn't need boron.

That notion started to change when research nutritionist Forrest H. Nielsen, Ph.D., and his USDA colleagues conducted a study to assess boron's effects on the bones of 12 postmenopausal women. The volunteers, who ranged in age from 48 to 82, were first put on a low-boron diet for 17 weeks. They got only a quarter of a milligram of the mineral a day in their food. (That's not terribly hard to do. Many Americans eat a low-boron diet every day.)

After the boron level in the bodies of the women was assured to be low, they were given a 3-milligram daily boron supplement. Throughout the study, the women's urine was tested to see if calcium, phosphorus, and magnesium were passing out of their systems. Excessive excretion of those minerals, which are crucial to bone integrity, can be a tip-off that our skeletons are being demineralized and weakened.

After just eight weeks of the higher boron intake, the amount of calcium being lost was cut by 40 percent. Losses of magnesium, and in some cases phosphorus, were also reduced.

But more exciting to Dr. Nielsen was the fact that boron doubled the levels of certain hormones. "These steroid hormones are thought to be very important for maintaining bone and calcium status," he told reporters. "In fact, estrogen-replacement therapy is currently the only proven treatment for osteoporosis."

None of this means that everybody concerned about the health of their bones should begin taking a boron supplement. For one thing, the study involved only 12 women and has not been confirmed by further testing. So the results must still be viewed as very preliminary. For another thing, large doses of boron can be toxic.

The Boron Moral

The lesson to be learned is the Principle of Nutritional Prudence: To take advantage of any possible benefit from a food factor that hasn't yet been shown to be beneficial (and in large doses can even be harmful), try a diet already proved to be healthful that also contains the unproven food factor. As it turns out, vegetables, fruits, and nuts tend to be high in boron. Broccoli, prunes, dates, raisins, almonds, peanuts, and soy-meal are particularly good sources. Meat has only negligible amounts. And all these foods can be part of a sensible low-fat, high-fiber, high-carbohydrate diet, which science says may help protect against heart disease, high blood pressure, cancer, and more.

By following such a diet, you'll be doing your health a big favor for a number of proven reasons. If the boron/bone connection pans out, you'll have another good reason. If it doesn't, you're still way ahead.

Counteracting Cataracts, Cancer, and More with Vitamin E

Vitamin E may really help our bodies withstand the ravages of time, toxins, and disease. That's the powerful suggestion coming from a conference of scientists who reported on their latest research. Their findings, presented here, show vitamin E's wide range of possible protective talents: in eyes and lungs; in brain cells damaged by Parkinson's disease; in chronic skin ulcers; in plaque-prone arteries; and in the body's infection-fighting immune system.

First, a Word about Antioxidants

Vitamin E's most important role, it appears, is as a potent antioxidant. Antioxidants protect against damage caused by oxidation. We can't live without oxygen, of course. But just as exposure to oxygen causes iron to rust and butter to turn rancid, it can wreak the biological equivalent in your body, rusting out cell membranes.

The villain in this process is something called a free radical. Understanding what a free radical is practically requires an advanced degree in chemistry. But for those of you who really want to know, this is as simple as we can make it: A free radical forms when a molecule somehow comes up with an odd number of electrons.

This can happen in a lot of different ways. But often this odd-electron phenomenon occurs when oxygen molecules rob other molecules of electrons.

Free radicals are created every minute, right in our bodies. All we have to do is breathe or run around the block and we're drawing electron-robbing molecules of oxygen into our systems. Normally, free radicals don't pose much of a problem. They're captured and inactivated by the body's own army of antioxidants. Trouble arises when free radicals outnumber antioxidants. That happens with aging (when the body's antioxidants dwindle) or exposure to pollution, cigarette smoke, and other toxins (which contain more free radicals than the body can handle).

Unchecked, free radicals roam the body, robbing other normal molecules of electrons (in effect, creating more free radicals) and causing the kind of cell damage we associate with oxidation.

That's why antioxidants are so important—and why researchers are so intrigued with the potential of vitamin E. Vitamin E is the body's principal fat-soluble antioxidant. That means where there's fat in the body—in blood lipids, the fatty sheaths on nerve fibers, or in any cell membrane—vitamin E is on free-radical patrol.

Only recently are researchers beginning to note the important implications of this on a wide variety of medical concerns.

Combating Cataracts

Most cataracts associated with aging occur when the normally clear, gelatin-like cells of the eye's lens are damaged, allowing tiny droplets of fat to leak out. Like dirt on a camera lens, these particles reflect and scatter light, blocking vision and giving the eye a distinct milky look.

Exposure to ultraviolet (UV) light is thought to be a major cause of cataracts. The light promotes oxidative damage to the cells of the lens. Many animal studies have been done on antioxidants and cataract formation over the past 20 years. In some, supplemental vitamin E helped slow (or prevent) the formation of cataracts in animals exposed to UV light.

The results of a recent survey conducted at the University of Western Ontario, in London, Ontario, suggest that vitamin E may also help prevent cataracts in people. There, researchers asked 175 people with cataracts about their intake of supplemental vitamins and compared their responses with those of a group of people of the same age and sex without cataracts.

The researchers found that people free of cataracts had taken significantly more supplemental vitamins E and C (another antioxidant) than those with cataracts. (They averaged 400 international units of E and 300 to 600 milligrams of C daily.) Those who took vitamin E alone were half as likely to have developed cataracts as those not taking it. Those who took both E and C had only one-third as many cataracts as those who took neither vitamin (*Annals of the New York Academy of Science*).

Of course, there are many unknown factors that may have contributed to these results. So it's difficult to say for certain how great an impact the supplements had. Still, it's a first step in realizing a potential link.

"This information could have a large impact on the incidence of cataracts in older people," says James Robertson, D.V.M., who conducted the study. Right now, approximately half of all of people age 75 or older have cataracts.

Next on Dr. Robertson's agenda? Hopefully, a long-term study to see if an "antioxidant cocktail" of vitamins E, C, and carotenoids like beta-carotene can help stop the formation of cataracts.

Postponing Parkinson's Disease

Parkinson's is a nervous-system disease that produces shaky hands and a shuffling gait. It's triggered by damage to movement-controlling brain cells found deep in the center of the brain. These cells produce a chemical, dopamine, that's essential for the brain to send messages to muscles. As the cells die and dopamine levels drop, muscle control suffers.

Unfortunately, no one knows what causes the brain-cell damage that provokes Parkinson's. But now, some researchers believe that it may be due, at least in part, to oxidation and free radicals.

To test this theory, Stanley Fahn, M.D., director of the movement disorder group at Columbia University, put several of his early-stage Parkinson's patients on megadoses of vitamins E and C.

Dr. Fahn was looking for clues that these two antioxidants might help slow the progression of the disease and thereby postpone initiation of drug therapy. (Levodopa, the drug of choice for Parkinson's, has undesirable side effects with long-term use.)

The results of his study? The 17 patients he has followed since 1984 were able to go 2½ years longer than another physician's patients who were not taking vitamins E and C before their symptoms required levodopa treatment.

Also, at the University of Medicine and Dentistry of New Jersey, researchers compared 81 Parkinson's patients (average age 65) with a sibling of the same sex and similar age without the disease. They were asked about the likelihood of having eaten any of 17 foods between the time they married (for most, around age 25) and age 40. Three foods were correlated with an absence of Parkinson's: nuts and seeds (sunflower seeds and walnuts topped the list), salad oil or dressing, and plums. Nuts, seeds, and oils are rich sources of vitamin E. Plums are only a fair source, but they are one of the best fruit sources of vitamin E (*Archives of Neurology*).

In another study, 14 Parkinson's patients who reported taking vitamin E daily for an average of seven years, in doses ranging from 400 to 3,200 international units, were compared to a similar group not taking vitamin E. When rated for severity of 41 signs and symptoms, including tremors, rigidity, slowness, walking and balance, the vitamin E users were found to have significantly fewer symptoms than nonusers.

"This evidence does seem to indicate vitamin E may help prevent Parkinson's and reduce its severity," says researcher Stewart Factor, D.O., of Albany Medical College. "But it's important to keep in mind that the studies were small." For firmer evidence, he's waiting for the results of a five-year study of 800 Parkinson's patients from around the country that's currently under way.

Curbing Cardiovascular Disease

Not all blood fats are created equal. There's good cholesterol (carried in high-density lipoproteins, or HDL) and there's bad (carried in low-density lipoproteins, or LDL). We know that HDL somehow ushers cholesterol out of the body, which is good, and LDL deposits cholesterol on the artery walls, which is bad. But we're still trying to understand the hows and whys.

Some researchers theorize that an early step in the formation of artery-clogging plaque is the oxidation of LDL cholesterol. Oxidized LDL cholesterol seems to trigger a complex reaction that leads to the buildup of fatty streaks on artery walls.

The question, then, becomes: Can vitamin E help prevent artery-clogging plaque? At least in animals, the answer is yes. When monkeys on high-cholesterol diets were given supplemental vitamin E, plaque formation slowed, compared to monkeys on the same diet without vitamin E supplements.

In another study, researchers at the University of Graz, in Austria, found that each LDL particle contains eight to ten antioxidant molecules, including six of vitamin E (and four carotenoids). These few molecules have the task of protecting about 1,000 polyunsaturated fatty acids in a single LDL particle from oxidation. But they can do only so much. Higher blood levels of vitamin E mean fewer free radicals.

What does this mean for someone worried about heart disease? It's too early to say with any certainty. "But this and other studies raise the possibility that the amount of vitamin E in blood and blood vessels may be a factor in determining how rapidly you develop atherosclerosis," says Lawrence Machlin,

Ph.D., director of Hoffmann-LaRoche's clinical nutrition department.

Improving Immunity

As we age, our ability to ward off infection gradually weakens. Our immune system's infection-fighting white blood cells become sparse, and those left are less capable of doing their job of destroying invading viruses, bacteria, or cancer cells. That's why cancer and other diseases become more common.

Some experts believe that age-related immune-system failure may be the result, in part, of a lifelong accumulation of oxidative damage to white blood cells (and to the progenitor stem cells that produce white cells).

In animals, supplemental vitamin E helps protect these cells from oxidative damage. It appears to enhance the ability of white blood cells to engulf and destroy bacteria, to control the production of biochemicals that cause inflammation, and to boost T-helper cell activity (cells that help other cells in destroying invading agents).

Now, for the first time, there's evidence vitamin E may do the same in humans.

Researchers at Tufts University/USDA Human Nutrition Research Center on Aging worked with 32 healthy older people. For one month, half the group took 800 international units of vitamin E a day; the other half received blank look-alike pills (placebos). Then blood samples were analyzed for several measures of immune response. Higher levels of certain biochemicals indicated immune function had improved.

Cells were better able to communicate among themselves (called cell-mediated immune response), which meant they could do "on-site battle coordination." A certain type of white blood cells, called T-cells, were also secreting more of a biochemical, interleukin-2, which stimulates them to divide and multiply.

We still don't know the proper dosages to produce optimal results, or more important, whether these effects can be sustained over time, says researcher Simin N. Meydani, D.V.M., Ph.D., of Tufts. But this is exciting stuff, nonetheless.

Healing Skin Ulcers

People with circulation problems often develop phlebitis, blood clots in the veins of their legs or arms. The clots cause limbs to swell, as stagnant blood leaks through vessel walls into surrounding tissues. The blood damages skin cells (even leaking into the upper layers of the skin), so most people with deep vein clots develop skin ulcers. The ulcers are treated with skin grafts, but blood circulation is often so poor the grafts slough off.

Researchers at Presbyterian-University Hospital in Pittsburgh knew from animal studies that skin cells were dying because excess blood oxidized fats in skin-cell membranes. They also knew that giving animals injections of antioxidant drugs helped skin cells to live.

So testing vitamin E as a treatment seemed a logical next step. Half of a group of 20 people with vein clots were started on 400 international units daily of vitamin E a few days before their skin grafts; the other people were not supplemented. The vitamins were continued for 14 months after the grafts. At that time, both groups were compared. The skin grafts in all of those getting vitamin E were healthy; but in the nonsupplemented group, every one of the grafts had broken down.

"These results were so dramatic that I now recommend vitamin E to every skin-graft patient I treat," says Sai Ramasastry, M.D., the study's main researcher. "None of my patients developed any side effects from this treatment." (Check with your doctor, though, before taking high doses of vitamin E, especially if you're on anticoagulant drugs.) His next step? To see if vitamin E can prevent skin ulcers from occurring in the first place, making skin grafts unnecessary.

Good News for a Bad Habit

Cigarette smoke contains numerous chemical catalysts that can trigger oxidation in living cells. So smoking enhances oxidative damage in the lung cell membranes. And it can hurt blood cell components as they pass through the lungs. That may be how two of smoking's worst consequences—cancer and heart disease—begin.

A study from Scotland offers preliminary evidence that vitamin E shields lung cells and red blood cells from such damage. (It's already been shown to lessen smoke-induced cell damage in animals.)

The study included 20 smokers and 20 nonsmokers, who took either 1,000 international units of vitamin E or a placebo daily for two weeks. At the end of that time, their blood was analyzed for its ability to withstand the kind of oxidative damage that occurs during exposure to cigarette smoke. The blood cells of smokers taking vitamin E were less likely to be damaged by that exposure.

"It will take years more to find out if additional vitamin E does indeed reduce smokers' risks for cancer and heart disease," says Garry Duthie, Ph.D., the study's main researcher.

Getting Your Vitamin E

What do you need to know before acting on any of this information?

First, keep in mind that these studies are preliminary; more research needs to be conducted before scientists are willing to give general guidelines for vitamin E supplementation. Nevertheless, many of the researchers we interviewed for this article do take vitamin E and recommend it to their patients. As cataract researcher Robertson puts it, "If someone in my family asked me, I'd say there is no guarantee vitamin E will prevent cataracts, cancer, or any other disease. But at these levels, there are also no known risks."

The levels of vitamin E used in the studies—generally between 400 and 800 international units per day—far exceed the Recommended Dietary Allowance of 12 to 15 international units. But, even at these high dosages, none of the participants in any of the studies cited here suffered adverse effects of the vitamin E supplementation. The vitamin can have a potentially dangerous blood-thinning effect, however, in some people (like those on anticoagulant drugs and those with vitamin K deficiency). If you have a medical problem, check with your physician before taking vitamin E supplements. And never substitute nutritional therapy for proper medical care or for a well-balanced diet.

Foods rich in vitamin E include sunflower seeds or oil, sesame seeds or oil, almonds or almond oil, canola, soy or corn oils.

Head Off Heart Trouble with Magnesium

Nutrition researchers call magnesium the "forgotten" mineral. Forgotten because it's never been considered a nutritional heavyweight like calcium or iron. Forgotten because severe cases of magnesium deficiency are rare. And forgotten because even though up to 90 percent of us may fall short of magnesium (the average American consumes about 40 percent of the Recommended Dietary Allowance, or RDA), none of us seems the worse for it.

Or could we be mistaken? The symptoms of a mild magnesium deficiency are silent, yes. But innocuous? Maybe not, say some medical scientists. Their studies suggest that a magnesium shortage, even slight, may contribute to serious health problems, including high blood pressure, heartbeat disturbances, and heart attack.

It's known that severe magnesium deficiency—usually the result of severe malnutrition or lengthy intravenous or diuretic therapy—can produce a conglomeration of symptoms. Anorexia (loss of appetite). Nausea. Weakness. Personality changes. Muscle spasms and tremor. Even potentially deadly arrhythmias.

Beating Arrhythmias

Arrhythmia—a change in the time or force of heart rhythm—means different things to different people. For some, it can be a rapidly pounding heartbeat; for others, an occasional skipped beat. One healthy person in 20 has arrhythmias of no known significance. In recovering heart attack patients, though, such arrhythmias can be dangerous.

Cardiologists have long known that low potassium causes arrhythmias. They now estimate that low magnesium is the culprit in about 1 case in 1,000.

Unfortunately, ordinary blood tests usually detect only severe magnesium deficiencies. So, unless a patient hits rock bottom, the doctor may not prescribe magnesium. And this, magnesium researchers say, may be a mistake. Preliminary studies show magnesium quiets arrhythmias even when blood tests appear normal.

Danish doctors studied 130 heart attack patients with magnesium levels that were, on average, low but within normal range. Seventy-four patients received an ineffective placebo substance—sugar water. Fifty-six received magnesium. To prevent bias, neither doctors nor patients knew who got what. Almost half the patients on the placebo had arrhythmias; seven died. Less than one-quarter of those on magnesium had arrhythmias; only two died (*Clinical Cardiology*).

A similar study carried out in Israel corroborated those findings. Again, the patients' magnesium levels were low but, on the whole, fell within the normal range. Of 94 heart attack patients, 48 received magnesium and 46 took placebos. A day after hospital admission, 16 patients on the placebo had potentially lethal arrhythmias. Only 7 on magnesium did (*Archives of Internal Medicine*).

Cardiologists are not yet convinced magnesium helps everyone with arrhythmias. But they caution that patients on digitalis should be monitored for magnesium deficiency. People with low levels of potassium and magnesium are vulnerable to digitalis toxicity, which can lead to arrhythmia, apparently by further depleting potassium and magnesium.

If you take digitalis and experience arrhythmia, talk to your doctor. You may need your medication dosage and your body's magnesium and potassium levels checked.

Controlling Cholesterol

Heartbeat perfect...but plagued by artery-clogging cholesterol? Researchers say you may have another reason to think magnesium. Surveys show that people living in hard-water, high-magnesium areas have fewer plaque deposits than people living in soft-water or hard-water, low-magnesium (high-calcium) areas.

Animal studies support the high-magnesium/low-cholesterol link. Rabbits fed a low-magnesium, high-cholesterol diet tend to have high blood cholesterol. But rabbits fed a high-magnesium, high-cholesterol diet tend to have half the blood cholesterol of low-magnesium rabbits.

Furthermore, the low-magnesium rabbits usually have almost twice the heart disease of the high-magnesium bunnies (*Magnesium*).

Of course, people aren't rabbits, and low cholesterol buildup in high-magnesium-water areas may be due to something other than magnesium. But researchers seem fairly certain that future research will verify these findings. "Based on the existing evidence, I'd say we've got two possibilities," says magnesium researcher Burton M. Altura, M.D., Ph.D. "First, low magnesium intake may predispose us to heart attacks. Second, adequate magnesium intake may help prevent heart attacks."

Meanwhile, researchers have raised another possibility: Low magnesium increases the size of a heart attack—that is, the number of heart cells that die during the heart attack. Animals low in magnesium tend to accumulate calcium in heart cells. And during a heart attack, these cells accumulate still more calcium—enough to damage them, studies show.

"If this happens in humans, too, it means low magnesium makes you more likely to die if you have a heart attack," says Sherman Bloom, M.D., of the University of Mississippi, author of some of these studies.

Link to High Blood Pressure

New studies also suggest low magnesium is linked to hypertension, a major risk factor for heart attack and stroke.

At Harvard Medical School and Brigham and Women's Hospital, Boston, researchers looked at diet and blood pressure in 58,218 women. Magnesium intake, researchers found, had an inverse association with blood pressure: Women consuming little magnesium developed more hypertension than did women getting lots of magnesium (*Circulation*).

Other researchers examined diet and blood pressure in 615 Hawaiian men. Again, magnesium intake had an inverse association with hypertension (*American Journal of Clinical Nutrition*).

Dr. Altura offers a theory that may explain the association. Hypertension sometimes results from a spasm of blood vessel muscles. Such a spasm may be a product of magnesium deficiency, he says.

Likewise, says Dr. Altura, getting enough magnesium may reduce blood pressure. Magnesium is a muscle relaxant, and it may relax blood vessel muscles enough to reduce or prevent hypertension, he theorizes.

If you're taking diuretics (which are, ironically, prescribed to control high blood pressure), you should be especially cautious. Cardiologists and magnesium researchers agree that drugs like chlorothiazide (Diuril), other thiazide-based diuretics and the more potent diuretic furosemide (Lasix) deplete magnesium. If you're taking one of these diuretics, consult your doctor. For some patients, it may be appropriate to switch to a milder diuretic, such as amiloride (Moduretic) or spironolactone (Aldalactone), which may help retain magnesium.

A Magnesium Miscellany

Researchers are pursuing hints about magnesium's effect on many other conditions. Some think low magnesium causes thymus gland lymphoma—cancer—in some animals.

Links between low magnesium and cancer in humans are less clear and more controversial. In any event, cancer patients shouldn't increase magnesium intake except under a doctor's care. Magnesium stimulates protein synthesis, and the most rapidly synthesizing cells are cancerous.

Magnesium deficiency may play a part in diabetes. Uncontrolled diabetes as well as insulin therapy may lead to magnesium loss. Also, deaths from diabetes seem to increase in areas where magnesium in drinking water is low (*Lancet*).

Does magnesium deficiency contribute to diabetic illnesses? Does diabetes produce magnesium deficiency? Scientists don't know. Until they do, diabetics' best bet is the American Diabetes Association's nutritional guidelines, which include such high-magnesium foods as whole grains and beans.

Other research has focused on pregnancy. In 1987, a 6,000-woman study found significantly lower blood magnesium in pregnant women than other women (*Journal of the American College of Nutrition*).

This past year, a study of 568 pregnant women found those on magnesium less likely than those on placebos to have premature babies. Babies of magnesium-supplemented mothers were less likely to need intensive care after delivery (*British Journal of Obstetrics and Gynecology*).

What to Do

The final verdict on magnesium is not in yet. This mineral has been extensively studied for 30 years—not long in scientific terms. Questions about it will likely persist decades more.

Although it's less common than magnesium deficiency, too much magnesium can also make trouble, stopping reflexes, respiration, and eventually, the heart. Normally, our kidneys dump excess magnesium in urine. In people with failing kidneys, though, a seemingly innocent quantity of certain antacids or laxatives, either of which may be high in magnesium, can be an overdose.

This much is certain: Unless you have failing kidneys, you can't go wrong getting the RDA of this often-forgotten mineral. For men, that's 350 milligrams per day; for women, 300 milligrams; for pregnant or lactating women, 450 milligrams.

Getting your daily dose of magnesium may be surprisingly easy. If you're lucky enough to live in a high-magnesium/hard-water area, you're probably already getting adequate levels of the mineral in your drinking water. Just be sure, if you have a water softener that removes minerals, that it bypasses the cold-water tap.

Mineral water, despite its name, seldom has much magnesium.

No matter what kind of water you drink, you can get plenty of magnesium from food. In general, a varied diet rich in fruits, vegetables and whole grain cereals, legumes, and unprocessed (coarse) flours is all you need to reach the RDA.

(Processing of foods, especially flours, can result in magnesium loss of 80 to 90 percent.) For most people, getting the RDA of magnesium is enough to prevent any problems. But if you have a condition that may be affected by magnesium, or you take digitalis or diuretics, talk to your doctor.

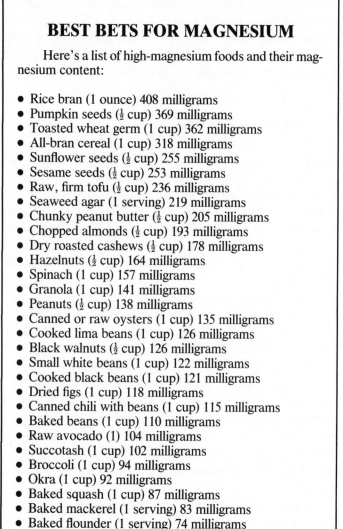

BEST BETS FOR MAGNESIUM

Here's a list of high-magnesium foods and their magnesium content:

- Rice bran (1 ounce) 408 milligrams
- Pumpkin seeds ($\frac{1}{2}$ cup) 369 milligrams
- Toasted wheat germ (1 cup) 362 milligrams
- All-bran cereal (1 cup) 318 milligrams
- Sunflower seeds ($\frac{1}{2}$ cup) 255 milligrams
- Sesame seeds ($\frac{1}{2}$ cup) 253 milligrams
- Raw, firm tofu ($\frac{1}{2}$ cup) 236 milligrams
- Seaweed agar (1 serving) 219 milligrams
- Chunky peanut butter ($\frac{1}{2}$ cup) 205 milligrams
- Chopped almonds ($\frac{1}{2}$ cup) 193 milligrams
- Dry roasted cashews ($\frac{1}{2}$ cup) 178 milligrams
- Hazelnuts ($\frac{1}{2}$ cup) 164 milligrams
- Spinach (1 cup) 157 milligrams
- Granola (1 cup) 141 milligrams
- Peanuts ($\frac{1}{2}$ cup) 138 milligrams
- Canned or raw oysters (1 cup) 135 milligrams
- Cooked lima beans (1 cup) 126 milligrams
- Black walnuts ($\frac{1}{2}$ cup) 126 milligrams
- Small white beans (1 cup) 122 milligrams
- Cooked black beans (1 cup) 121 milligrams
- Dried figs (1 cup) 118 milligrams
- Canned chili with beans (1 cup) 115 milligrams
- Baked beans (1 cup) 110 milligrams
- Raw avocado (1) 104 milligrams
- Succotash (1 cup) 102 milligrams
- Broccoli (1 cup) 94 milligrams
- Okra (1 cup) 92 milligrams
- Baked squash (1 cup) 87 milligrams
- Baked mackerel (1 serving) 83 milligrams
- Baked flounder (1 serving) 74 milligrams
- Cooked oatmeal (1 cup) 56 milligrams

New Roles
for Protein Building Blocks

Anyone who remembers the relentless wasting away of baseball player Lou Gehrig knows the deadliness of the disease that bears his name. No one knows what causes amyotrophic lateral sclerosis (ALS). It is known, however, that this incurable disease involves the deterioration of nerves in the spine and brain stem that control muscles, and that death comes when its victims can no longer swallow or breathe.

But new scientific evidence offers hope that there may be something that helps slow this killer's course. It's neither lasers nor drugs nor scalpels—it's amino acids.

They're commonplace pieces of protein that we get in our food every day of our lives. Amino acids activate many of the body's metabolic processes—from building muscles to producing the chemicals that make our brain work. Most people get all the amino acids they need, in the right balance, by eating only a few ounces each day of protein-rich foods. But now more than ever, researchers are using them therapeutically—that is, in doses larger than you'd get in food—to try to fight not just ALS but several other serious conditions as well.

In the war on ALS, the weapons are three amino acids called leucine, isoleucine, and valine, usually given in large doses. It's known that outside the nerve cells of ALS victims, there's a buildup of another amino acid, glutamate.

While nerve cells do need glutamate to fire off messages, too much can be toxic. It can actually kill the cells. The amino acids leucine, isoleucine, and valine, however, have been shown to stimulate the breakdown of glutamate. So researchers in the Department of Neurology at Mount Sinai School of Medicine in New York City theorized that leucine, isoleucine, and valine might prevent the buildup of glutamate.

They studied 22 ALS patients who, when they entered the study, were able to walk and had no other disease. For a year, half the group received the three amino acids. The other half received inactive look-alikes (placebos). The patients were evaluated every three months by doctors who didn't know which substance the patients were taking.

At the end of the year, the two groups were compared. Those taking placebos had muscle deterioration considered normal for the disease. Five had lost their ability to walk. In contrast, the amino acids group had lost much less muscle strength. Only one had become wheelchair-bound. In a number of muscle-strength tests, the amino acids group did about four times better than the placebo group (*Lancet*).

"These results are very encouraging," says Andreas Plaitakis, M.D., the study's main researcher. "This treatment, however, is still experimental. We need to learn much more about it before it's safe to recommend." He's now organizing a nationwide study funded by the Muscular Dystrophy Association.

Experts stress the fact that the amino acids used in this research are really acting as drugs, and that no one knows yet what the nutrients' full effect on the body might be. No ALS patient should try any amino acids without a doctor's supervision.

The other research on amino acids is also in its early stages—and has stirred just as much interest in their disease-fighting potential.

Saving Muscles after Injury

Intravenous protein solutions are standard treatment for people who've been badly burned or injured. By supplying amino acids, the solutions help prevent the body from breaking down protein in muscles and organs to rebuild its injured parts. One amino acid, arginine, seems to outshine the others in this regard. In animals with fractures, diets supplemented with arginine and glycine (another amino acid) reduced the loss of protein from the muscles by 40 percent, researchers at Rutgers University in New Jersey found. And researchers at Einstein Medical School in New York City found that, after moderate surgery, people who got an extra 15 grams of arginine a day had a 60 percent reduction in protein loss compared with patients who did not get the supplement.

What does this mean right now for someone recovering

CAN AMINO ACIDS BUILD BIGGER MUSCLES?

You may have seen amino-acid mixes on the market that promise to help pump up muscles fast. (Weight-loss and immune-boosting formulas are also being sold.) None of these amino products have Food and Drug Administration approval, and there's very little scientific evidence to back up their claims. Yet some weight lifters swear by the muscle-building mixes as well as certain individual amino acids.

The weight lifters place their highest hopes on the amino acids arginine and ornithine, claiming that the nutrients help beef up muscles and are safer than steroids.

But there's little research in this area. What we do know is that arginine, injected into the bloodstream, does stimulate the release of growth hormone, a substance that makes cells multiply faster. (Arginine injections are actually used to detect growth-hormone problems in children.) Ornithine, an amino acid that can be formed from arginine, may prove to be an even more potent growth hormone stimulator.

But things aren't quite so simple as some bodybuilders might like them to be. First, the bodybuilders take oral supplements of amino acids, not injections. During digestion, changes in composition could eliminate the amino acids' effect on growth hormone. Second, if oral amino acids are indeed found to stimulate growth hormone, the effect could be dangerous. It could cause the same kind of abnormal bone growth seen in a disease called acromegaly. Or it could promote the development of diabetes. The long-term effects of these amino acids truly are unknown. Researchers in this field warn: User beware!

from surgery or injury? "Some intravenous solutions now contain more arginine than previously," says Adrian Barbul, M.D., a pioneering arginine researcher. "But this research doesn't mean people should take amino acid supplements after some trauma."

Most doctors say that until more studies are done, the best bet for people who have been injured or undergone surgery is simply to make sure they eat a well-balanced diet that contains recommended amounts of vitamins, minerals, and protein.

Lifting Depression

The dark shadows of serious depression may be more a function of physiology than psyche, researchers now think, with malfunctions or deficiencies in brain chemistry to blame. Antidepressant drugs can help correct the problem. They increase the production of neurotransmitters, chemicals that send messages throughout the brain and help us stay alert and active. Or they prevent "reuptake" (absorption) of neurotransmitters so that more of the chemicals are available to the brain. Or they make nerve cells more sensitive to neurotransmitters (by increasing "receptor sites" on nerve cells).

Now some researchers think that certain amino acids may be able to manipulate neurotransmitters to beat depression. They suggest that neurotransmitter deficiencies may cause depression, and if neurotransmitter building-blocks (certain amino acids) are provided, the mind may regain its healthy outlook.

One promising antidepression amino is tryptophan, which is known to raise brain levels of serotonin (an important brain neurotransmitter that elevates mood) in animals. It's one of the better studied and more commonly used amino acids and the only one with Food and Drug Administration approval for treatment of insomnia. (Some antidepressant drugs also raise serotonin levels. Tryptophan in large doses and antidepressants also seem to improve sleep and relieve chronic pain.)

In studies, tryptophan alone seems to be only a mild antidepressant, a better cure for the blues than for suicidal sadness. It may work best when used along with antidepressant drugs, says Lawrence H. Price, M.D., director of the Clinical Neuroscience Research Unit at Yale University. Researchers there found that 15 of 21 depressed patients who had improved while taking antidepressant drugs relapsed when they were depleted of tryptophan. They recovered when they got adequate amounts of tryptophan.

L-phenylalanine, an amino acid used by the body to make

the neurotransmitter phenylethylamine, is also sometimes used to treat depression. It is said to give an amphetamine-like boost in mood and energy. Although some forms of phenylalanine do seem promising for some kinds of depression (particularly bipolar, or manic depression), more research is needed before recommendations can be made, says Hector Sabelli, M.D., of Rush Presbyterian/St. Luke's Hospital in Chicago. Dr. Sabelli has done studies that show that L-phenylalanine lifted depression in some manic-depressive patients.

Dr. Price and other researchers feel that certain amino acids may indeed help some depressed patients, especially those who haven't responded to several different antidepressants. Dr. Price believes that amino acids should be used in conjunction with drugs. (Some doctors prefer to use them alone.) He and other doctors caution that amino acid therapy is not a substitute for medical evaluation and treatment for depression, including medication and psychotherapy if you need it. Depression can be caused by many factors.

The Prevention Perspective

The experts agree: Until we know more about the impact of supplemental amino acids on the body, no one should use them as a treatment, at least not without a doctor's supervision. Why? Because to work, amino acids usually have to be used in large amounts, which have unknown toxicity. They compete with other nutrients in the body and may need to be taken with or without other foods. They may increase the requirements of other nutrients, like vitamin B_6 and magnesium. And you may be taking drugs that make amino acids build up to toxic amounts in your body and your brain. If you have a health problem you think may be helped by amino acids, discuss it with your doctor.

Big News about B_6

So what's to know about an already well known B vitamin whose U.S. Recommended Daily Allowance (USRDA) is a minute 2 milligrams?

Nothing much, unless you count recent scientific research showing B_6 to be a promising or proven treatment for several health problems. Or unless you include the fact that B_6 affects practically every major system in the body. (It helps manufacture amino acids, the building blocks of cells; concoct neurotransmitters, the messengers of the central nervous system; break down carbohydrates into glucose, our chief source of energy; create the oxygen-carrying portion of red blood cells; even manufacture antibodies to fight infection.) Or unless you factor in the very real possibility that you're lacking in this vital nutrient.

Judge for yourself. Here's our distillation of 12 of the most important, most useful B_6 facts:

Fact #1: Most People Don't Meet the USRDA for B_6 • In fact, only slightly more than 19 percent of the population gets the recommended 2 milligrams. More than 60 percent consume 1.6 milligrams or less. The people with the lowest intake: women and the elderly.

Serious B_6 deficiency, fortunately, is rare. (Symptoms include a kind of skin rash, lack of muscle coordination, depression, and anemia.) But it's people with mild deficiencies who have some researchers worried. "Moderately B_6-deficient people may have problems we don't recognize, or even know to look for," says James E. Leklem, Ph.D., a professor of human nutrition at Oregon State University. The smartest course is to get the recommended amount.

Fact #2: Certain Drugs Can Cause Deficiencies despite Adequate Intake of B_6 • They do this not by destroying B_6, but by blocking its use. The most common B_6 bashers are:

- Theophylline, for asthma
- Penicillamine, for rheumatoid arthritis
- Isoniazid, for tuberculosis
- Hydralazine, for high blood pressure

If you're taking any of these medications for several weeks or longer, you may need to consume extra B_6.

Fact #3: B₆ Can Beat a Serious Kidney-Stone Disease • Oxalic acid, a substance found in many foods, is harmless to most of us. But in some people it contributes to kidney stones, especially those with a rare genetic disorder called hyperoxaluria. These people excrete abnormal amounts of oxalic acid into their urine. Over time, this can cause calcium buildup—and kidney stones.

B₆ reduces the amount of oxalic acid that is excreted, preventing new stone formation. B₆ can't dissolve stones that have already formed, and it's not a cure for any other type of kidney stones. But it's a standard therapy for this disorder.

Fact #4: B₆ Counteracts Too Much Estrogen • Taking a lot of estrogen can actually cause B₆ deficiency. The older high-estrogen birth control pills made some women depressed and moody. A supplement of 15 to 20 milligrams of B₆ easily reversed these symptoms. Most newer, low-estrogen pills have little effect on B₆ levels, but now there's another area of concern: estrogen-replacement therapy for postmenopausal problems or osteoporosis. Experts say that women who undergo these treatments would be wise to include more B₆-rich foods in their diet.

Fact #5: B₆ Has Become a Promising Treatment for "Hopeless" Autism • Autism is a mysterious and tragic behavioral disorder. Autistic children seem to live inside their heads, cut off from the rest of the world. Sometimes they can become violent or self-abusive. Many don't speak. Autism affects 4 or 5 children out of every 10,000. Some of these children become more "manageable" with drug therapy, but they don't really lead normal lives.

Several researchers in the United States and in France, however, have reported remarkable behavioral improvements in autistic children who are given B₆. According to Bernard Rimland, Ph.D., director of the Institute for Child Behavior Research in San Diego, the effective dose is about 300 milligrams of B₆ per day. This dose, he says, must be accompanied by the USRDA of magnesium and other B vitamins for maximum benefit with minimal side effects.

In one study, three children spoke for the first time after the B_6 treatment began. Special-education teachers documented behavioral improvements in some children's class records, and noted renewed problems that corresponded to the end of treatment. Nothing remarkable there—except the teachers weren't told that the students were on a new therapy. Parents, who obviously were aware of the therapy, rated the changes they noticed. Out of 318 autistic children, 43 percent were rated better-behaved, 52 percent remained about the same, and only 5 percent got worse. These figures beat the standard drugs, which have "got worse" rates of anywhere from 16 to 51 percent. Most drugs improve only 20 to 30 percent of patients. According to Dr. Rimland, the B_6-and-magnesium treatment has virtually no significant side effects. While not generally accepted by physicians, the B_6/magnesium treatment is gaining a following as a safer alternative to drugs.

Fact #6: B_6 Can Help Some Cases of Carpal Tunnel Syndrome • An important nerve passes through a narrow opening in the bones of the wrist, the carpal tunnel. Injury or overuse can put pressure on the nerve, causing numbness and/or pain. People who must perform repetitive tasks using their wrists—typists, assembly-line workers, and others—are at greatest risk. There are about half a million new cases of CTS each year.

"B_6 can ease the pain for many CTS sufferers," says Allan L. Bernstein, M.D., chief neurologist at Kaiser-Permanente Medical Center in Hayward, California, "But those who have normal B_6 levels usually won't respond to vitamin therapy." And other CTS experts agree.

Dr. Bernstein has successfully treated hundreds of CTS patients with a combination of B_6 supplements and wrist splints. His patients take 150 milligrams of B_6 per day. The vitamin apparently starts working after 8 to 12 weeks. (Some earlier studies that suggested B_6 was ineffective ran for only six weeks.) The dosage is maintained for a few months, then the patient is gradually weaned off treatment with lower doses. Many people have avoided wrist surgery with this treatment.

(All experts agree, however, that CTS can be a serious problem and should be treated by your doctor.)

Fact #7: B₆ Calms Seizures • For people with a rare vitamin-dependency form of epilepsy—about 1 out of 1,000 epileptics—the only treatment is megadoses of B₆. Without this treatment, they're subject to seizures. For all other types of epilepsy, though, B₆ is of no use.

Fact #8: Scientists Are Testing to See If B₆ Can Boost Immunity • One of the most exciting new areas of B₆ research is in immune function. The most intriguing study so far comes from Oregon State University. Eleven healthy subjects (aged 65 to 81) were given 50 milligrams of pyridoxine per day for two months. When their blood samples were tested in a lab, the infection-fighting white blood cells called lymphocytes had increased their activity significantly. Lorraine T. Miller, Ph.D., a professor of nutrition and one of the authors of the study, says that the next step will be to duplicate this experiment and to measure immune function in the test subjects.

Fact #9: Too Much B₆ Can Hurt You • For years, nutritionists thought that only fat-soluble vitamins like A and E, which are stored in the body, are dangerous in high doses. B₆ is one of the water-soluble (not stored) vitamins, which were thought to be nontoxic in virtually any dose. But now there are reports of a few people suffering nerve damage with B₆ doses as low as 200 milligrams per day. Some who took 1,000 to 2,000 milligrams per day were disoriented and even partly paralyzed. If caught early, the symptoms can be reversed by simply stopping the high doses. Now many experts agree that the maximum safe dose for B₆ is probably somewhere below 200 milligrams per day. But it's better to err on the side of safety and not exceed 50 milligrams of B₆ per day without a doctor's supervision.

Fact #10: B₆ Isn't One Nutrient, but Three • It's three related compounds: pyridoxine, pyridoxal, and pyridoxamine. All are easy to absorb and use, but you'll encounter them in different places: pyridoxine in most vitamin supplements, and pyridoxal and pyridoxamine in meat.

Fact #11: The World's Best No-Fat Natural Source of B$_6$ is the Banana • It's a B$_6$ treasure trove, providing one-third of the USRDA with 0.7 milligrams per serving. Walnuts, peanuts, wheat germ, whole grains, avocados, potatoes, and blackstrap molasses are other good plant sources. Meat, fish, and poultry are also fine sources of B$_6$, but you have to be careful of the fat. Half a breast of roasted chicken (without skin) contains 0.51 milligrams of B$_6$—more than one-quarter of the USRDA. Six ounces of salmon contains 0.37 milligrams, and six ounces of broiled sirloin provides a hefty 0.76 milligrams.

Fact #12: You Can Get an Entire Day's Worth of B$_6$ in a Single Meal—Breakfast • That's because a lot of fortified cereals contain up to 100 percent of the USRDA. Check the side panel of the box for exact information.

Protecting and Restoring Your Good Health

Folk Cures on the Medical Frontier

For folk healer and pharmaceutical researcher alike, the whole earth is a medicine chest. Nature, traditionally, has yielded some of the most potent weapons against disease. From the bark of a Peruvian tree came quinine, the first known treatment and cure for malaria. From the purple foxglove came digitalis, a drug that makes a weak heart heartier. And from willow bark came the early form of aspirin, salicin. All of these were folk remedies before modern science "discovered" them.

Varro Tyler, Ph.D., professor of pharmacognosy at Purdue University, estimates that one-quarter of today's drugs are derived from natural sources, and about 10 percent actually have their roots in folk healing. In fact, natural substances continue to be fertile ground for serious pharmaceutical research, and many may become the wonder drugs of tomorrow. Here's a selection of the latest crop of promising nature cures to undergo scientific scrutiny.

Feverfew Spells Fewer Migraines

This aromatic herb has long been a folk cure for migraine headaches. Now a recent study at the University of Nottingham, in England, gives it scientific backing. Researchers studied 60 migraine sufferers. Half received capsules con-

159

taining ground feverfew leaves and half received inactive capsules for four months. Then the groups switched for four
months. The researchers found a 24 percent reduction in the
number of headaches while the people were taking feverfew.
Vomiting was also reduced. So was the severity of the attacks.
And there were no significant side effects (*Lancet*).

In test-tube studies, feverfew inhibits the release of serotonin, a brain chemical that constricts blood vessels. Scientists
suspect migraines may result when blood elements called
platelets release excess serotonin.

Here's a Honey of a Healer

Results of a three-year clinical trial at University Teaching
Hospital, in Calabar, Nigeria, suggest that unprocessed honey
may heal wounds when more conventional dressings and antibiotic treatments fail. In 59 patients treated for wounds and
ulcers, honey was effective in all but one case. Topical application kept sterile wounds sterile until they healed, while infected
wounds became sterile within a week. This study also showed
that honey can be used to remove dead tissue from persistent
wounds, helping some patients avoid skin graft or amputation
(*British Journal of Surgery*).

Honey is slightly acidic and absorbs water, which may
account for its ability to reduce swelling in wounds, the researchers say. It also contains an antibacterial agent called
inhibine.

Mutant Fungi May Yield Anticancer Drugs

Two newly developed strains of fungus yield large
amounts of toxins called trichothecenes, potential cancer
fighters. By themselves, trichothecenes kill both normal and
cancerous cells. But when combined with monoclonal antibodies, proteins custom designed to zero in on cancerous cells,
they may become potent anticancer drugs. The mutant fungi
were developed by Marian N. Beremand, Ph.D., a geneticist in
the Agricultural Research Service of the U.S. Department of
Agriculture. Her research could increase the number of different trichothecene compounds available. "Cancer researchers

may wish to select one kind of trichothecene that works best for a particular type of cancer," she says.

Chinese Weed Chokes Malaria

A centuries-old Chinese treatment for malaria has inspired international research on the healing properties of a weed, *Artemisia annua*. Laboratory and animal studies show that arteether, a drug derived from the weed, is effective against the malaria parasite. The active ingredient is a molecule called qinghaosu. Scientists are now attempting to produce a derivative of qinghaosu that will be more potent and easier for the body to assimilate (*Journal of Medicinal Chemistry*).

Amphibians Yield Antibiotics

A scientist's observation that frogs stay infection free while swimming in bacteria-laden water may have important implications for victims of cystic fibrosis, burns, and infectious diseases. Michael A. Zasloff, M.D., Ph.D., chief of human genetics at the Children's Hospital of Philadelphia, discovered—and was later able to synthesize—two slightly different strains of a powerful new antibiotic produced by the glands in a frog's skin. The antibiotics, which Dr. Zasloff calls magainins, are the first chemical defense other than the immune system to be found in vertebrates. Dr. Zasloff thinks humans may produce a similar chemical. He suspects that cystic fibrosis, a genetic disease characterized by bacterial infection of the lungs, may be caused by a defect in this system.

Broiled Cactus Stems Diabetes

Mexican herbologists have long advised clients with diabetes to eat the stems of the nopal cactus. Recently, Mexican researchers found that 12 of 16 subjects who ate broiled nopal cactus stems had a significant drop in their blood sugar (glucose) levels within an hour. Glucose levels continued to decline for the next 2 hours. By comparison, diabetics eating broiled squash did not benefit. The researchers think something in the cactus may improve the cells' ability to use glucose, and that it may be useful in managing diabetes (*Diabetes Care*).

Ginkgo Breakthrough Fans New Research

Asians have relied on extracts of the fan-shaped ginkgo leaf since 3,000 B.C. to heal a wide variety of ills. Now the active ingredient, ginkgolide B, has been synthesized in the lab for the first time by Elias J. Corey, Ph.D., a Harvard professor. As a result, stepped-up research in this country and in Europe could lead to new treatments for asthma, toxic shock syndrome, and circulatory and kidney disorders. Ginkgo extracts even offer promise as a safer alternative to the drugs now used by organ-transplant recipients.

How ginkgolide B works is not yet known. One theory is that the compound interferes with a chemical in the body called PAF, or platelet activating factor. PAF has been implicated in graft rejection, asthma, and other immune disorders.

Five
Bone-Building Strategies

By George L. Blackburn, M.D., Ph.D.

Some of us are lucky enough to be born into a family with strong bones. Good genes, it seems, can give us an edge against osteoporosis, a bone-thinning condition that often develops in later years. But good genes can't guarantee protection. By the same token, a family history of osteoporosis can predict who's a more likely candidate for thinning bones. Bad genes alone won't do you in. Bad habits, however, can—regardless of your family's health history.

Don't set yourself up for a shattering fall; take the time, now, to evaluate your own health habits. If you answer yes to any of the following questions, your bones may be coming up short.

Do You Assume
You're Getting Enough Calcium?

You may be wrong. When scientists screen people for nutrient deficiencies, they usually find calcium among the top three that most people are lacking. (The other two are iron and vitamin E.) And since bone continually is broken down and new bone formed from the calcium you eat, it's important that your intake remain consistently high throughout life. If you deprive your body of dietary calcium, the withdrawals will exceed the deposits. Result: excessive bone-weakening. It takes a conscious effort to ensure your calcium intake is adequate for healthy bone. If you ignore calcium, it will go away.

Women who don't eat dairy products are particularly susceptible to shortages. But anyone can fall short, if he or she is not careful. In general, men should consume at least 800 milligrams of calcium daily; premenopausal women should get at least 1,000 milligrams daily, and postmenopausal women should consume at least 1,200 milligrams daily (the equivalent of four 8-ounce glasses of milk).

You can achieve healthy calcium levels by eating about three servings daily of calcium-rich foods, especially low-fat dairy products like nonfat and low-fat yogurt, 1 percent fat and skim milk, and low-fat cheeses. If you don't eat dairy products, it's considerably harder to get enough calcium. Although there are nondairy foods, such as sardines, tofu, and chick-peas that are calcium-rich, you might also need a calcium supplement. But don't take supplements greater than 1,000 milligrams without the advice of a physician. (Too much calcium can be a problem for some people—about 10 percent of the population—who have certain kidney and parathyroid disorders.)

If you aren't sure whether your diet provides enough calcium, it's a good idea to write down everything you eat and drink (particularly the portion size) for four to seven days, and bring that food diary to a registered dietitian for evaluation.

Do You Guzzle Soft Drinks?

You may be flushing calcium from your bones. Colas and certain other carbonated drinks get their bubbles from phosphorus, containing the mineral phosphate. Phosphate, along with calcium, is in your bones in a 1 to 1 ratio. The trouble is, if you pour in too much phosphate, your body will excrete it—and when phosphate leaves, it takes calcium with it. Where does it get the calcium? From your bones.

So try to limit yourself to two servings of phosphate-containing sodas each day. Better yet, check the labels and choose carbonated beverages that don't contain phosphates. (Carbonated mineral waters do not contain phosphate.) And whenever possible, ask yourself whether a glass of low-fat milk might satisfy your thirst just as well.

What worries me the most is that children are the target of many soft-drink ads. Yet those under ten, whose bones are actively growing, are weakening their bones, and may even suffer impaired bone development if they overindulge in soda and don't consume enough calcium-rich foods.

Are You a Big Meat Eater?

Excess protein, particularly animal protein, may bind with calcium in the digestive tract, preventing absorption. Most Americans consume way too much protein anyway. By limiting yourself to two modest, 3- to 6-ounce servings of meat each day, you'll meet your protein requirements with little interference in calcium absorption.

Are You Eating
Too Much of a Good Thing?

Spinach and soybeans (two nutrient-rich foods), as well as cocoa, are high in oxylate, a chemical compound that has been shown to interfere with calcium absorption. (By the way, there usually isn't enough cocoa in hot chocolate to significantly block the absorption of the calcium in the milk.) That's not to say you should eliminate these foods from your diet. Just don't overdo.

Incidentally, it is an unfortunate fact that high-fiber foods, which can help regulate the bowels and reduce blood cholesterol, can also interfere with calcium absorption. The health benefits of a high-fiber diet are so significant, however, that you shouldn't cut back for calcium's sake. And as long as you get the daily amount of calcium suggested above, you needn't worry about the relatively small effect of fiber.

Are You a Step Saver?

To build healthy bones, you need to get up on your skeleton and move it. Exercise makes bones stronger, just as it makes muscles stronger. For bone health and general fitness, at a minimum you should be moving vigorously for 200 minutes a week; ideally, 400 minutes. That doesn't mean a formal exercise program for all those minutes! It can include everything from climbing stairs to vacuuming your apartment.

Also, it's a myth that bone-strengthening exercise should be a high-impact, bone-jarring activity like running. Walking can do the trick. So can hiking and cycling. The gentlest exercise, swimming, also helps strengthen bone, but probably not as much as walking.

Remember, too, that it's never too late to invest in strong bones. Even if you're near or past menopause, when bone-thinning is likely to accelerate, increasing calcium intake and exercise level may make a difference. At any age, you can prevent excess calcium loss, and if you're on a comprehensive exercise program and careful diet, it may even be possible to restore lost bone.

Push Your Pressure Down

When it comes to high blood pressure, every point counts. Studies show that if you're hypertensive, every little incremental rise in blood pressure corresponds to a jump in your risk of heart disease and stroke. So anything you can do to nudge your blood pressure down—if only a few points—is all to the good.

To that end, here is a smorgasbord of 29 techniques you can use right now to counterpunch hypertension. Experts point out that such "lifestyle strategies" have in many cases helped people to either cut back on their antihypertensive medication or drop their blood pressure into the safety zone.

Is every one of these strategies guaranteed to lower your blood pressure significantly? Not at all. Everybody is different: What works for someone else may not work for you. And though science has declared some of the techniques highly effective in reducing chronic high blood pressure, others aren't as highly rated. Some of these may push blood pressure down, but only temporarily. Or they may simply be the latest untested-yet-safe proposal for making a dent in your hypertension. The point is that if you're really serious about lowering high blood pressure, they're all worth a try, especially since every little bit of pressure-lowering helps.

So the idea is to try as many of these strategies as possible (under your doctor's supervision and as adjuncts to any medical treatment you may be undergoing). There's every reason to believe that a lot of the techniques will have a cumulative effect. They're more likely to be effective, however, if you have mild hypertension—a systolic reading (the first number) of 140 to 159 or a diastolic reading (the second number) of 90 to 104. But even higher pressures may respond to some of these strategies. Typically, though, medication is the first and most prudent therapy for people with severe hypertension—systolic of 160 or higher, or diastolic of 115 or higher.

1. Lose Weight • If you're overweight, this is one of the most potent antihypertension lifestyle changes you can make. It has a proven impact: On the average, people can lose one point off both their systolic and diastolic blood pressures for every two pounds they drop.

2. Eat Fish • Preliminary studies have suggested an association between eating fish or fish oil and lower blood pressure. Researchers theorize that it's the omega-3 fatty acids in ocean fish (such as mackerel, tuna, and salmon) that could somehow be counteracting hypertension. The experts' recommendation: Dine on fish at least two or three times a week.

3. Go for a Walk • Research shows that regular aerobic exercise (walking, cycling, swimming, and the like) may lower blood pressure four or five points. How much exercise does it take? Most of the studies reporting decreases in blood pressure in hypertensives had people working out 30 to 60 minutes three times a week. (You have to work up to this level slowly, though, and with your doctor's blessing.)

4. Say When • Over the long haul, consuming more than two mixed drinks (1 ounce of alcohol each), two beers, or two glasses of wine a day can raise your blood pressure. The danger of lower amounts is unclear, but experts are unanimous in their recommendation: Limit the booze. Alcohol abuse has been called "the most common cause of reversible hypertension."

5. Watch the Fat • The evidence is far from conclusive, but some research suggests that intake of saturated fats (prevalent in red meat, many dairy products, and other foods) may be linked to rises in blood pressure. And polyunsaturated fats (prevalent in certain vegetable products like safflower and corn oil) seem to lower it. A growing mass of evidence suggests that monounsaturated fats, predominant in olive oil and a few other foods, may provide the same benefits. So experts are advocating a prudent course. First, lower your total fat intake to less than 30 percent of calories. Then keep the saturated fats to a minimum (no more than one-third of total fat), and favor the monos and polys.

6. Find Your True Blood Pressure • Some people with high blood pressure are believed to have "white-coat hypertension." Their blood pressure rockets only when it's taken in their doctor's office. So before you make a commitment to blood pressure medication, have your pressure measured over a full day with a portable unit. (Your doctor may loan one out.) Or have your blood pressure measured several times in a variety of settings.

7. Don't Salt the Water • Water softeners replace calcium and magnesium with sodium. So use your softener, just don't hook it up to the tap water used for cooking and drinking.

8. Eat a Baked Potato • A baked potato with no added sodium has a powerful "K Factor," says potassium expert George Webb, Ph.D., associate professor of physiology and biophysics at the University of Vermont Medical College. It has 130 times more potassium (chemical symbol: K) than sodium. Lack of potassium has been associated with an increase in blood pressure. And some researchers feel that the key thing is to maintain a 2-to-1 or 3-to-1 ratio of potassium to sodium in your diet. In general, fresh fruits and vegetables have far more potassium than sodium. Top choices: beans, rice, fresh fruits, and grains. (Check with your doctor. Some people with certain kidney diseases can't tolerate extra potassium.)

9. Beware the Pill • Oral contraceptives raise blood pressure slightly in most women and are estimated to cause high blood pressure in about 5 percent. So if you want to use oral contraceptives, ask your doctor about using a preparation with low estrogen/progestogen content. Low-dose formulas are less likely to have a pressure-raising effect.

10. Steam It • Boiling vegetables leaches away a good part of their potassium and magnesium (another mineral that may be linked to reduced blood pressure) and allows sodium to be picked up more easily by the food. It's even worse, of course, if you add salt. So as part of your own antihypertension campaign, microwave, steam or bake your food. Stir-frying is okay, but use oil sparingly.

11. Pet Your Dog • Or your rabbit. Or your cat. Any animal that's soft and cuddly. Some researchers suspect that interacting with a pet may lower blood pressure, at least temporarily. "The minute you start talking to and petting your dog, your blood pressure goes down and stays down during the interaction," says Aline Halstead Kidd, Ph.D., professor in psychology at Mills College in Oakland, California. In a 1986 survey, some 20 percent of the doctors polled thought hypertensive patients could benefit by going to the dogs. "The point is, human-to-human interactions make certain demands. A pet allows you to interact with another living being that makes no demands and loves you without regard to anything." It's important that the animal be yours, Dr. Kidd says. Meeting a strange pet can entail the same cautious social minuet as when you meet another person.

12. Look at Fish • "Anything that holds your attention so you're looking and listening but not thinking and worrying reduces blood pressure transiently," says Aaron Katcher, M.D., a psychiatrist at the University of Pennsylvania. "And this could be from watching a fireplace, taking a walk in the park, going bird-watching, or watching fish in an aquarium." Based on studies of other relaxation techniques, Dr. Katcher believes that doing any of these things for 15 minutes twice a day may be an effective treatment for some people with mild hypertension.

13. Do Your Own Stress Test • Though it's possible to be perfectly calm and still have hypertension, or have normal blood pressure and be a nervous wreck, some people do react to stress with at least a temporary rise in blood pressure. And scientists suspect that stress plays a still-unknown role in chronic hypertension. So to find out for sure if stress is boosting your blood pressure, test yourself. Buy a home blood pressure monitor and have it calibrated by your physician or pharmacist (otherwise it may be off by as much as 30 points). Your doctor can show you the proper sitting position and technique for taking your pressure. Then take your blood pressure before, during, and after a stressful activity. This way you'll know if the stressful event is affecting your blood pressure and whether you should avoid it. Good news: Not all stressful or exciting situations have an effect.

14. Live with Less Sodium • Not everyone with high blood pressure is affected by dietary sodium (the main ingredient in salt), but most are. And you may be one of them. Excess sodium will cause sodium-sensitive people to retain more fluid, which can raise blood pressure. Hormonal changes may also contribute by constricting blood vessels. Unfortunately, there's no easy way to determine who's sodium sensitive. But most of us consume far too much sodium and could stand to cut back. So experts say reduce your total daily sodium intake to 1,500 to 2,000 milligrams—the amount you'd find in 1 teaspoon of salt. Even modest reductions may be enough to enable some people to reduce or even eliminate their hypertension medication.

15. Check Your Water • Your largest source of sodium, if you're on a sodium-restricted diet, could be a surprising one— your drinking water. It doesn't necessarily taste salty. In a 1981 study, 42 percent of the nation's water supply exceeded the Environmental Protection Agency's (EPA) recommendation of 20 milligrams of sodium per liter. Check your water sodium level with your local water supplier or the EPA.

16. Measure Often • The regular measuring of blood pressure over time seems to help some people nudge their pressure down. One possible reason: If you're aware of your blood pressure, you may take steps (perhaps even subconsciously) that may help, such as not dousing your baked potato with salt. Or reacting more serenely to stress.

17. Enjoy a Good Laugh • A hearty laugh causes a small and fleeting decrease in blood pressure. Even more important, laughter is a great way to relieve stress and anger. Go to a funny movie. Be with people who make you laugh, rather than those who debate. The long-term effects of laughter on blood pressure are unknown, but certainly there are no negative side effects to laughing.

18. Use Diet Pills with Caution • Many diet pills, both prescription and over the counter, contain a substance that's a mouthful—phenylpropanolamine (PPA). PPA is believed to depress the part of the brain that controls appetite. But in some people it can also raise blood pressure, among other possible side effects.

19. Select Fast Foods Wisely • Many fast foods are loaded with sodium and fat. A McDonald's Big Mac has 950 milligrams of sodium. A Burger King Whopper with cheese has 1,164 milligrams of sodium, which can by itself exceed the recommended amounts for those on sodium-restricted diets.

20. Keep an Anger Diary • Both habitually holding anger in or lashing out without trying to solve a problem can lead to transient—and possibly chronic—increases in blood pressure. Keeping track of your anger in a diary, however, helps you identify and understand the causes of your anger. Your diary should monitor what made you angry, what you did about it, how you felt at the time and later. Then you can reflect and develop strategies for defusing anger constructively.

21. Relax from Head to Toe • Progressive muscle relaxation is a proven technique for relieving stress. Sit or lie in a comfortable position and tense and relax the muscles of your body in sequence. Start by clenching your fists for 3 or 4 seconds, concentrating on how the tension feels, then relax your hand muscles, letting go of the tension.

Try this tensing/relaxing sequence for all major muscles—those in your neck, shoulders, back, arms, abdomen, buttocks, thighs, calves, and feet. Ideally, you'll learn to relax these muscles without tensing them first. Try this exercise for 10 minutes, twice a day.

22. Smell a Slice of Apple Pie • Preliminary research suggests that certain scents—particularly spiced apple—may nearly double any blood pressure benefits of quiet relaxation. One theory is that apple pie can bring back pleasant associations with holidays. The research is too inconclusive to say that a given odor will nudge your own blood pressure down. But if you want to test the notion, try a fragrance you find particularly appealing.

23. Watch for "Hidden" Salt • Cured meats, such as bacon, hot dogs, and sausage, are high in sodium and fat. Many (but not all) canned soups are high in sodium. So are some brands of canned tuna, prepared pancakes, some TV dinners, and regular soy sauce. So become a label reader when you grocery shop.

24. Listen to Music • There's no hard scientific data yet, but some music-therapy experts think that tuning in to tunes may help lower blood pressure. But what kind of music? Heavy metal? Ugh. The experts suggest that the best tunes are of the soothing kind—quiet, nonvocal, slow, with predictable rhythms.

25. Check Your Medication • Propranolol, a common antihypertensive that slows heart rate, may limit the cardiovascular benefits of a workout, according to a study from the University of Vermont School of Medicine. One of these benefits is decreased blood pressure. (The benefits of the drug itself, of course, remain intact.) So if you exercise and are taking propranolol, ask your doctor about switching to another blood pressure drug.

26. Talk to Yourself • You can learn to respond more calmly to a stressful or anger-provoking situation by talking your way through it beforehand. For example, let's say you have to meet with someone who often irritates you. Instead of saying to yourself, "I'm going to lose it when he acts like a jerk," say "There's no reason to automatically assume that he'll get on my nerves. I'm going to stay relaxed. I won't get angry."

27. Work as a Team • Blood pressure experts say that you're more likely to stick with any antihypertensive regimen if you enlist the whole family in the effort. Some suggestions: Do exercises that other family members can enjoy with you, like walking and bicycling. Don't keep food in the house that one person can eat but another cannot.

28. Douse That Cigarette • Studies show that smokers seem to get less benefit from the pressure-lowering drug propranolol. Also, though smoking itself doesn't seem to raise blood pressure over the long run, it can damage the cardiovascular system and make the consequences of having high blood pressure worse.

29. Watch What You Chew • Chew this over: Smokeless tobacco often contains large amounts of sodium for flavor and also to help the body absorb nicotine.

Power Living for Prime-Timers

With baby boomers pushing past 35, a major segment of the American population is hitting prime time. This is life at its fullest. Active. Changing. Settled. Unsettling. You can thrive on it!

To begin, "prime" yourself with smart health habits. The truth is, age is no gauge of physical stamina and mental smarts. Body/mind fitness is. And today it's the people in the middle—the so-called sandwich generation—who are grasping health with both hands.

Here, then, is a host of reassuring new facts and today's hottest tips for high health in the middle years. The "prime" focus: supercharged nutrition; fitness you can feel; weight-management measures you can live with; and more. Plus, there are five profiles of prime-timers who've put themselves squarely on the fast track of health.

Supercharged Nutrition

Reverse "Nutritional Aging" • Hurrah: Nutritionists confirm that in the middle years you don't go through some kind of metabolic time warp in which your body requires more and more nutrients just to get by. But you do have to watch out for some sly, age-related changes in your nutrient intake. Government surveys reveal that many people aged 23 to 50 have alarmingly low intakes of certain nutrients. At least a third of the men surveyed weren't getting enough vitamins A and B_6, calcium, and magnesium. One-third to three-quarters of the women lacked all these nutrients plus vitamin C, folate, and iron.

Two suspected causes of the deficits: reduced-calorie diets that cut nutrients along with calories, and low-fat/low-cholesterol diets that restrict the intake of certain foods containing some scarce nutrients.

One solution is to eat more foods that pack multiples of the elusive vitamins and minerals. Some good prospects are broccoli (for vitamins A and C and calcium), sunflower seeds (for vitamin B_6, folate, and iron), beans (for vitamin B_6, folate, magnesium, and iron), salmon and white-meat chicken (for vitamin B_6 and folate), and cantaloupe (for vitamins A and C).

Another option for some people is taking supplements. "I always encourage people to meet their nutritional needs through diet," says registered dietitian and nutrition consultant Jo-Ann Heslin. "But getting adequate nutrition this way isn't always possible—especially for people on restricted diets. For them, taking a daily, balanced multivitamin is a good idea."

Be a Smarter Coffee-Lover • Coffee-drinking habits ingrained in earlier years tend to continue and sometimes accelerate through the middle years. If you can keep a lid on your consumption—at, say, one to two cups a day—you're okay.

But if you find your intake on an upward track, there may be good reason to reverse the trend. Reason one: The tannins in coffee (and tea) can play mean games with vitamins and minerals. "Tannins at mealtime may reduce your body's ability to absorb nutrients from the food, throwing even a balanced diet out of whack," says nutritionist Liz Applegate, Ph.D., nutrition director of the adult fitness and cardiac rehabilitation program at the University of California, Davis. "So if you really enjoy a good cup of coffee or tea, drink it between meals."

Reason two: Some research has found an association between coffee drinking and cholesterol levels in the blood. A recent Finnish study of over 12,000 people, for example, showed an association between heavy coffee consumption and high blood cholesterol levels. In the people aged 45 to 64, the highest cholesterol levels were found in those drinking four to six cups of coffee a day. Other studies have failed to find a coffee/cholesterol connection. But until the issue is settled, some experts are saying go easy on the java.

"Until we know more, I recommend limiting your intake

to two cups of tea or coffee (decaf included) per day," Dr. Applegate says. "And avoid these beverages altogether if you have a family history of heart disease, are overweight, eat a high-fat diet, or never exercise."

PRIME-TIME MAKEOVER: JUDITH PAIGE, 50

What advice would you give to a white-haired woman of 50 who wants to abandon a successful, hard-won career in order to seek her fortune as a fashion model?

Judith Paige says that her friends' response was, "Go for it!" And she did. About a year ago, she was a chief nutritionist at a Boston hospital. But she had a yen to model and a hunch that she could represent people her age in a positive way. "Yes, it was audacious," she laughs. She put her finances in order, arranged for some part-time consulting work, and signed up with a modeling agency. In one dizzying year, she's succeeded beyond her wildest dreams.

This isn't the first successful midlife career change for Judith Paige. At 35, a homemaker and divorced mother of two daughters, she returned to school to begin a grueling five-year training program in nutrition. At 40, she became a registered dietitian.

Returning to school and work wasn't easy. But, contrary to warnings, she found that her age and experience were pluses. "When I was applying for nutritionist jobs, everyone else was 20. But I wasn't afraid to write my age in my resume: I would say, 'I have raised a family; I have skills in personal relationships and life.' It's an advantage. I would even think, 'This isn't fair to everyone else. Too bad. They can go to a plastic surgeon and have wrinkles implanted!' "

Paige credits 20 years of yoga with giving her much of her mental and physical stamina and grace. "The way you feel after you do yoga is really terrific. It gives me a lot of strength in my body, and that translates into psychological strength."

Outmaneuver "Metabolic Slowdown" • You say your eating and exercising habits have remained constant over the years, but your weight hasn't? Are you blaming those "love handles," "saddlebags," and other middle-age parcels of pudge on a slowed metabolism? Well, you may have a point. The body's metabolism slows slightly as we age. "The slowdown is only about 2 percent per decade," says Heslin, "accounting for a weight gain of about 3 or 4 pounds in that time."

Compensating for a 2 percent slowdown in metabolism requires a 2 percent decrease in calorie intake (assuming your activity level remains constant). If your diet consists of 1,800 calories per day, a daily 2 percent cutback is 36 calories—equivalent to a teaspoon of butter, or 2 teaspoons of sugar, or less than one chocolate chip cookie. No big deal!

Beat the "Big Three" • Prime-timers, take note. Three of the biggest—and sneakiest—sources of excess calories (and excess girth!) are:

• Alcohol. It's liquid calories and little nutrition. Seven ounces of wine, for example, contain 306 calories—about the same as a slice of Boston cream pie. A Manhattan packs 233 calories—about as much as an eclair. To get around such numbers, you can try halving your intake, going for reduced-calorie wine and beer, or substituting sparkling waters and other nonalcoholic beverages.
• Dessert. You love it, and you don't have to leave it to avoid caloric overload. Just scale down your desires, say nutritionists—a smaller slice of pie, a cupcake instead of a slab of chocolate cake, a small dish of ice cream rather than a banana split.
• Fat. Avoid this—unless you want to wear it, say obesity specialists. They point out that dietary fat is converted to body fat much more readily than carbohydrates or protein. So if you're going to cut calories, cut the ones from fat first.

Get Off the Yo-Yo • By the time you reach your middle years, you may have lost a fast 20 pounds—one dozen times. The result of all this gaining/losing/gaining (the old yo-yo syndrome) is that each time you try to drop a few pounds, it just gets harder, and harder, and—forget it.

One thing that each gain/lose cycle does is reduce your total muscle tissue and increase your body fat. And since fat burns fewer calories than muscle, each bout of dieting just makes maintaining or losing weight more difficult.

To break through the yo-yo syndrome, experts advise 40 minutes of moderate exercise a day (to speed up your metabolism and increase muscle mass) and a healthy high-carbohydrate, low-fat diet.

There's no need to starve yourself, says weight-loss authority George L. Blackburn, M.D., Ph.D., of Harvard Medical School.

The fact is, extreme low-calorie diets downshift your metabolism—exactly what you don't want to happen. So eat up. Just pare down your diet to the essentials—whole wheat bread, pasta, rice, fruits and vegetables, skim milk, fish, and skinless chicken. No mixed dishes. No goulash. No lasagna.

Body Conditioning

Work with Weights • Muscles and tendons are like the shrubs and bushes in your yard: They wilt not because of age, but from neglect. One study, conducted at Tufts University, found that men in their sixties and seventies were able to increase their muscle size by an average of 11 percent and their strength by a staggering 170 percent with just a 12-week weight-training program.

"A new study we're doing on strength-trained men has found that, to our surprise, lifting weights really burns off the calories," says Tufts researcher Carol Meredith, Ph.D. "It seems to be an energy-expensive exercise."

S-t-r-e-t-c-h • If your toe touching isn't what it used to be, hang loose. Inflexibility, like loss of muscle tone, is not a sign of impending middle age. "Some flexibility may be lost in the middle years," says Dr. Meredith. "But it can be conserved to a considerable extent." Los Angeles physical therapist Randy Ice explains: "Connective tissue has a property of shortening if you don't use it. The more inactive you are, the shorter these

PRIME-TIME MAKEOVER: PHYLLIS KAHN, 51

There's a joke among Minnesota state legislators, says Representative Phyllis Kahn, that the job "provides a salary, plus all you can eat." But it was no laughing matter when, after her first session as an elected official, she gained about 10 pounds. "It was the combination of a lot of sitting, irregular meals, and fund-raisers and receptions." Kahn felt that she had no time for exercise; and year after year, she added pounds during legislative sessions.

Then, at age 40, her life changed dramatically. "We got a new dog that I thought needed more exercise," Kahn chuckles. "So I started running with the dog. The first time, I got halfway around the block and I thought I was going to die. I figured that anything that makes me feel this rotten this quickly has got to be good for me!"

Joking aside, Kahn took on the challenge of running with the same determination she brings to her work on the House floor. Within a year, she was participating in races and had run her first marathon. Since then she's completed some 25 marathons and holds a few state speed records for her age group. Nonetheless, she insists, most mornings she runs "really slowly." "I don't have that trained athlete's urge to push myself, which is probably better in the long run."

Kahn insists that she is hardly unique among her friends in taking up athletics in midlife. "I know more women in their forties and fifties who are born-again jocks!

"I ride with a women's bicycling group," she notes. "I describe it as the equivalent of my mother's and grandmother's canasta group. These are women in their forties and fifties whose children are grown, who have flexible schedules or are not working. Every Tuesday, we meet for lunch—but instead of going to lunch, we ride for 30 to 60 miles.

"I tell my secretary to try to keep my Tuesdays clear. Or I wear my bike shorts under my dress-for-success suit, and when it's time to go, I pull off my skirt, put on my bike shoes and—like Superman dashing out of a phone booth—I'm off to meet the group on the road!"

structures become, and the more difficult it becomes to do even routine things like gardening and lifting groceries out of your trunk. But if you stay active, you can stay limber. And you'll be less prone to back and muscle injuries than someone whose muscles are tight.''

Best bet: regular walking, combined with gentle stretching before and after.

Strengthen Your Abs • Strong abdominal muscles improve your posture and lower your chance of back injury. Best bet: bent-knee sit-ups.

Hang in There: Fitness Gains Can Be Yours at Any Age • The theory used to be that, beginning with middle age, every year costs you 1 to 2 percent of your aerobic capacity (a key indicator of endurance and fitness). According to that, in 20 years, you could lose as much as 40 percent!

Now a new study explodes that theory. It shows that, over 20 years, aerobic capacity declined only 12 percent in subjects exercising regularly. Two exercisers actually increased their aerobic capacity over the 20-year span.

Don't Succumb to "Lazy-Boy Spread" • You may think of it as "middle-age spread." But a new study shows that the amount of time spent exercising—not the amount of years spent living—is the most determining factor for excess body fat. The study, which compared men in their fifties and twenties, found that the more a man exercised, the lower his percentage of body fat—regardless of age.

Think "Consistency," Not "Intensity" • "Regular exercise can give you the equivalent of ten years' rejuvenation," says exercise researcher Roy Shephard, M.D., Ph.D., of the University of Toronto. "You don't need a particularly strenuous program either. You just need to be reasonably active."

Ice agrees. "If your goal is overall fitness and weight maintenance, your best strategy is to exercise at a comfortable level over a long period." Best bets: swimming, bicycling, rowing, and brisk walking. "We're currently conducting a

PRIME-TIME MAKEOVER:
TOM MONAGHAN, 51

Tom Monaghan's past reads like a rags-to-riches classic. Born in poverty and shunted from orphanage to foster home as a child, he went on to reach multimillionaire status the old-fashioned way: relentless hard work. "I put in 100-hour weeks tossing pizza in Ypsilanti, Michigan," he recalls. Today Monaghan is president of the Domino's Pizza empire and owner of the Detroit Tigers. Having "made it," he's got a new set of goals for his middle years: physical health and spiritual rejuvenation.

Mornings go like this: He wakes up at 5:45 A.M. Most days, he runs from 7:00 to 8:00, for about 6½ miles, "not breaking any speed records." He works out—floor exercises, Nautilus, and/or free weights—from 8:00 to 8:30. He attends Catholic mass till 9:00, then takes 20 minutes for personal meditation before beginning his business day.

It's time well invested, he says. He once weighed 30 pounds more than he does now. Also, "about eight years ago, I had lower back problems—my back muscles would just seize up on me. But I haven't had a lower back problem in three to four years."

As you might sense, Monaghan is a man who strives to implement his personal ideas and principles. He's ordered all the elevators in his company's four-story headquarters in Ann Arbor, Michigan, to be set to run as slowly as possible. "That's to encourage employees to climb the stairs," he explains.

A few years ago, Monaghan offered one of his franchise executives $50,000—yes, five-oh, oh, oh, oh—if he ran an entire marathon within a year. The executive did it, shedding 100 excess pounds in the process. Sure enough, Monaghan was standing at the finish line to present him with a giant-sized check. That stunt gave Domino's great publicity—in fact, most of the newspapers never got around to mentioning that the marathon was sponsored by a different food chain!

If there's a moral to Tom Monaghan's story, it's that good health means good business.

study on the effects of fast walking on middle-aged and older women," Dr. Meredith adds, "and we're finding it does increase physical fitness and decrease body fat."

Go for the Burn • Basal metabolic rate (the rate at which calories are burned to fuel the body's basic biological functions) does slow down with age—but just 2 to 3 percent every ten years after age 20. The bigger problem is that, as those decades roll by, we tend to eat more and exercise less, says Dr. Applegate. As a result, we gain fat and lose muscle, the body's most metabolically active tissue. Metabolism slows. The good news is that aerobic exercise can help you burn fat, build muscle and stoke your calorie-burning furnace all at the same time.

Cardiovascular Conditioning

Exercise to Your Heart's Content • According to a study of 3,100 men conducted at the University of North Carolina at Chapel Hill, getting in shape offers more heart protection than pushing back the clock 19 years. And conversely, lack of fitness is riskier than even smoking.

Exercise in Moderation • A University of Minnesota study showed that men with very low activity levels had a heart attack mortality rate of 24.6 deaths per 1,000 men; those with very high activity levels had rates of only 15.8 per 1,000. But those with moderate levels had the lowest rates, 15.4 per 1,000. Regular moderate exercise has been shown to lower high blood pressure and blood cholesterol, two major risk factors for heart disease.

Contraception

Continue Using Birth Control for a Full Year after Your Last Period • Hormonal changes that bring on menopause usually begin five or more years before menstruation ceases. (On average, menopause begins around age 50 or 51.) The last period can occur as long as 9 to 12 months after what seems to be the end of menses.

PRIME-TIME MAKEOVER: JANE BRODY, 47

When she was in her twenties, Jane Brody weighed a third more than she does today. "My present lifestyle evolved," she says, "and it evolved from knowledge—from having to confront, through the course of my work, the fact that the way I live can have a very dramatic impact on my health, and on my chances of living a long, healthy, and fulfilling life."

Brody, the award-winning medical writer for the *New York Times* and author of several health and nutrition best-sellers, is quick to admit her own lifestyle wasn't always so exemplary.

"I used to be a chronic starve-and-binge dieter," she recalls. "Now I'm careful never to skip a meal. It only makes me hungrier for the next meal and increases the likelihood that I'll overeat." If she should consume too much for lunch, she'll limit herself to a large salad and bread for dinner.

To be sure, her three daily meals are high in complex carbohydrates and very low in fat. Grains provide half of her protein and the rest comes from low-fat dairy products, poultry, fish, and small amounts of red meat. Her sweet tooth has abated in her middle years, she reports. When a craving does strike, she allows herself one or two moderately sweet treats a day, like a homemade muffin.

Brody says that making time for healthful home cooking while busy with a career and raising children (she's got 18-year-old twins) isn't as formidable as it sounds. Especially if you have a microwave. "I make stuff in large batches and freeze individual or family-sized portions. The microwave is a godsend, not to heat prepared dinners but to thaw and heat your homemade dinners!" To complement her healthy diet, Brody has gradually expanded her fitness pursuits beyond the biweekly tennis matches she used to play in her twenties. Nowadays she exercises for an hour to an hour and a half daily. "I have a varied exercise program—I run, walk, bike, swim, play tennis, ice skate, cross-country ski, and hike. Let's see," she laughs, "did I leave anything out?

"Once I made exercising a priority, it came ahead of other things. It comes way ahead of watching TV, which I almost never do." And she has no plans to slow down.

(continued)

PRIME TIME MAKEOVER—*Continued*

After all, "I just invested in new skates and cross-country skis. I have two excellent tennis rackets!"

In midlife, Brody says, her lifestyle has many pay-offs. For one thing, she credits her fitness regimen with the fact that she needs less sleep than she did ten years ago. "I sleep about 5½ hours a night. I used to sleep 6½. I sleep like I've been hit over the head with a brick—and then I wake up refreshed."

Also, she considers her exercise sessions—most of which she does early in the morning in Brooklyn's Prospect Park, near her home—as opportunities for spiritual rejuvenation. "I have seen more beautiful sunrises in New York than 99 percent of people."

Consider Barrier Methods First • Despite the high-tech options available, a diaphragm and other barrier contraceptives are still the recommended methods for the middle years. A condom, used together with contraceptive foam, is almost 100 percent effective with no dangerous side effects, for example.

Ask Your Doctor about the New Copper IUD • You could be a candidate if you're in a mutually monogamous relationship and have no prior history of pelvic inflammatory disease (PID). The T 380A (GynoPharma, Inc.) is 99 percent effective and—compared to IUDs of years past—is relatively safe. A poly-ethylene monofilament string minimizes the chance of bacteria wicking up into the uterus.

Ask about Low-Dose Birth-Control Pills • Although they are now an option for some women up to age 45, and possibly longer, they are not for everyone. Smokers and persons with diabetes, high blood pressure, or high cholesterol levels need not apply, says Dan Mishell, M.D., professor of obstetrics and gynecology at the University of Southern California School of Medicine, Los Angeles. But for other women, the newest oral contraceptives may be worth considering. Risks of heart attack and stroke—major complications with the old pills—have been reduced by as much as 80 percent with oral contraceptives containing less than 50 milligrams of estrogen. The multiphasics—which deliver just 20 to 35 milligrams of estrogen (less than one-fifth the amount of the earlier pills) and progestin (synthetic progesterone) in a combination designed to mimic nature—are considered the safest. Plus, there is now solid evidence that using low-dose pills provides long-lasting protection against ovarian and endometrial cancer. Ask your doctor about other risks and benefits.

Considering Sterilization? • Of the more than half-dozen techniques for sterilization, minilaparotomy is the safest and least expensive choice for women. Of course, vasectomy is even safer and less expensive!

Afraid You Might Change Your Mind? • Consider clip sterilization. It can be successfully reversed in almost 90 percent of cases.

Good Sex

Midlife Sex Can Be Better Than Ever • Women's sexual interest tends to peak in the late thirties or early forties, and midlife men tend to be better lovers. They have years of experience to fortify their bedroom savvy. And because mature males may take longer to become aroused and require more direct physical stimulation, they have to go slowly and savor the whole-body experience! Both partners now have a better chance to become fully aroused.

Talk and Touch • "These are the water and light a relationship needs," according to sex counselors Lorna Sarrel and Philip Sarrel, M.D. If slow sexual responses are misinterpreted as loss of desire, a negative cycle can result in which each member of the couple takes the blame. Communicate your feelings, needs, and doubts. In fact, the Sarrels recommend that you never let more than 24 hours go by without sharing some personal, meaningful worry, hope, idea, or feeling. Don't let small hurts smolder; talk about them. And touch at least every 48 hours—not just sexually, but with real body contact.

Men, Do Your Heart Good and Maximize Potency • Erections result from a rush of blood to the penis. So good sex depends on good blood circulation—one more reason to stop smoking, get plenty of exercise, and eat a low-fat, low-cholesterol diet!

Women and Men, Do Your Kegels • Kegel exercises strengthen the PC (pubococcygeus) muscle that stretches across the pelvic floor. Women typically practice Kegels to strengthen vaginal muscles after pregnancy. But men can benefit, too: A strong PC muscle can result in firmer erections, greater ejaculatory control, more powerful orgasms, and fewer prostate problems. To do Kegels, contract the PC muscle using the same motion you would to stop a stream of urine. Half your contractions can be brief; hold the other half for 3 to 5 seconds. Start with ten contractions a day and gradually work up to 50 or 100 a day.

Look for Lubrin at Your Drugstore • This nonprescription vaginal suppository is the most convenient lubricant. Lubrin lasts from 30 minutes to an hour. It dissolves rapidly and feels natural. Best of all, it's water soluble but not water based, so it won't evaporate and won't stain. It's also unscented, colorless, nonirritating, and nontoxic. It costs about $2.50 for five inserts.

Stay Sexually Active • Sexually active postmenopausal women continue to have healthy vaginas despite the absence of estrogen, and continue to lubricate as long as they remain active.

Consider Hormone-Replacement Therapy (HRT) That Includes Testosterone • Studies show that women receiving HRT consisting of testosterone and estrogen are twice as likely to be involved in a sexual relationship, report stronger interest in sex, and rate their sex lives as very enjoyable compared to women who receive estrogen alone.

PRIME-TIME MAKEOVER:
BILL LYONS, 50

Overweight and out of shape. That's how Bill Lyons describes his earlier years. "I had a paper route when I was a boy: that was it." Today he cycles about 100 miles a week. Twice a year, he participates in centuries, arduous 100-mile rides completed in one day.

Pretty good, especially when you consider that Lyons' life of fitness began just four years ago, at the ripe *middle* age of 46. That's when Lyons, who is president of a Los Angeles printing company, suffered a major heart attack. It struck at midnight, in a hotel room, while he was on a business trip in Nevada. "Ever go through a casino lying on a gurney? People think you're just another big loser," he jests.

But in fact, he almost lost it all. Lyons was rushed out of the hotel—past the casino in the lobby—and to a local hospital. There he underwent an angioplasty.

When he returned home, his doctors prescribed exercises on a treadmill, rowing machine, and stationary bicycle. "I progressed," Lyons says, "but I thought it was superboring."

Then someone told him about the Los Angeles-based SCORE Cardiac Cyclist Club, headed by physical therapist Randy Ice. Two months after the heart attack, he began cycling with the club, starting with a few miles each Saturday. He gradually increased his mileage, and today he's one of the stars of the club, pedaling 100 miles every week.

The rewards of the road have been many. "My weight is way down and I have a lot more energy," he boasts. "I just feel so much better for it. I never meet a hill I can't walk up."

What's more, as a result of his experience, his wife, who is 51, experienced a midlife turnaround, too. She's taken up cycling and lost weight. This summer, the couple will cycle through Italy—250 miles in nine days. His four children (including twin daughters, age 23) were similarly inspired. Lyons reports proudly, "One just ran a marathon, another is a triathlete, and all four are avid cyclists!"

Help for Menopause

Keep a Log of Your Hot Flashes • Note when they occur relative to your menstrual cycle. Also, chart your diet and stress level to see if there's any correlation. Some women find that caffeine, alcohol, hot soups, spicy foods, or heavy meals may provoke hot flashes. Stress also has been implicated.

Talk to Your Doctor about HRT • Sexual concerns aside, hormone therapy can help quell hot flashes and protect women from heart disease and osteoporosis. Two new methods of HRT include estrogen cream applied to the skin or inserted into the vagina, and estrogen implants beneath the skin, which release hormones continuously for about six months. Both methods reduce complications, such as elevated blood pressure and gallstones, that can arise with oral estrogen. Often estrogen is supplemented with progestin to counter estrogen's overstimulation of the uterine lining, which has been associated with a higher rate of endometrial cancer. Still, doctors do not recommend estrogen replacement to obese women or women with a history of breast cancer.

Healthy Relationships

Look for Signs of Burnout • Sudden job changes, unnecessary relocation, and the desire for new gadgets and toys are sometimes markers of marital burnout. Another clue is the amount of time spent watching television. "Television today is often called the electronic fireplace, but unlike a real fireplace, no talking or sharing goes on in front of it," says Paul Welter, Ed.D., author of *Counseling and the Search for Meaning.*

Beware of Boredom • "Boredom is the number-one cause of marriage burnout in the middle years," says Dr. Welter. "It occurs when a person feels that he or she knows everything there is to know about their spouse and explores no further."

Can You Think of One Really Interesting Thing Your Mate Said Last Week? • If you can't, you either don't listen as well as you could or you haven't learned to appreciate your mate's interests.

Share • Explore the world together and share in that sense of wonder and discovery. Cultivate friends you both can enjoy. "Sharing tasks is another good way to initiate discovery of each other," suggests Dr. Welter. "Chores often get segmented into solitary duties. Instead, make those mundane jobs—like painting the den or cleaning the garage—a joint effort."

Seed Questions • Ask your mate what caption was under his or her high school yearbook picture. What is his or her best memory from elementary school? The answers may reveal new facets of your mate's personality.

Job Transition

Change Jobs Only for the Right Reasons • "Ask yourself honestly if you're not trying to find a certain excitement and satisfaction in your job that in fact should be provided by your marriage," says Michael Nichols, Ph.D., author of *Turning Forty in the Eighties*.

Ready to Change Jobs? • Give it one last shot. Work harder, work smarter. If the thrill does not come back within three to six months, move on.

Attend to Your Interests before Attending to Your Bank Account • Although they are sometimes hard to separate, job satisfaction and multifigured paychecks are not the same thing. First, narrow your job search to positions that fit your interests. Then consider the dollar factor.

Consider Your Age Your Biggest Asset • It brings experience with it. Plus, the ability to solve practical problems tends to show an increase with age, says Steven Cornelius, Ph.D., associate professor of human development at Cornell University. Additionally, besides hard job skills, you've probably acquired a kind of second sense with regard to correct social maneuverings in the workplace.

Brainpower

Challenge Your Mind to Stay Sharp • IQ does not decline with age, says Mary Howell, M.D., director of the Kennedy Aging Project in Waltham, Massachusetts. Today a large body of data suggests that people who stay mentally active retain their IQs and may even improve them in the areas of information and vocabulary.

Don't Act Your Age • Put yourself in your child's shoes. Investigate. Discover. Play. Learn new skills. Take up a musical instrument or try your hand at a computer keyboard. You're never too old to grow. Take a cue from child-development experts.

Limit Your TV Viewing Time • "TV is one of the great thieves of mental acuity because it is a totally passive form of entertainment that makes no demands on the viewer," says Dr. Howell, both a trained pediatrician and gerontologist. Instead, tone your mental muscles with crossword puzzles and stimulating board games like chess or Scrabble.

Know You Can Conquer the World—Creatively Speaking • "While there is some evidence that creative productivity peaks in the early twenties, it may be due more to an abundance of energy and a conquer-the-world attitude rather than a higher abstract or cognitive intelligence quotient," says Dr. Howell. Two cases in point: Fyodor Dostoyevski wrote *The Brothers Karamazov* at age 58; Johann Strauss composed "The Blue Danube" at 41.

Don't Blame Memory Lapses on Middle Age • The rate at which we forget things already learned does not decline with age. Everyday memory lapses are usually the fault of poor memory techniques, says Robin West, Ph.D., author of *Memory Fitness over Forty*. With practice, she says, most people could boost their memory—some studies show by 50 percent.

Pay Attention • Quick, what's on the back of a $20 bill? You can't say you forgot because, chances are, you simply never noticed. If you can't remember where you put your keys, could it be you were setting down the groceries, humming a tune, and planning dinner at the same time? Force yourself to observe some minute detail concerning any object or event you wish to remember. You'll be surprised how fast your mnemonic mastery will return.

Clear Up Indoor Air Pollution

You probably already work hard to avoid the unwanted chemical by-products of twentieth-century living.

If you garden organically, you know that commonsense techniques can allow you to grow a bounty of food and flowers without synthetic pesticides and other substances that disrupt the ecological balance.

But what about your home? For the majority of Americans, closing the front door is no escape from air pollution. Study after study reveals that the quality of air indoors is often worse than the air outside. Even if you already avoid the use of pesticides and other indoor chemicals, you could still have a problem.

That's because the most common causes of indoor air problems are things that are difficult to perceive of as threats. They're the modern conveniences that we've come to take for granted: central air conditioning, gas appliances, home heaters—even carpeting.

But if smart gardeners can thwart crop-killing pests without resorting to the latest commercial "spray of death," you can certainly learn how to relax at home without inhaling a rogue's gallery of toxic substances.

Here's a quick look at some common indoor air problems and what you can do about them.

Air Conditioners

Indoor air is generally pretty good in the spring and early summer simply because most people open their windows fairly often. This action lets the bad air escape while the fresh air comes flying in. But when summer starts to swelter and air conditioners come on, more than cool air may wind up blowing into your home.

Stymied by the symptoms—thick mucus, endless throat clearing, fatigue, and confusion—that several patients were experiencing, Robert Jacobs, M.D., an associate scientist in the Department of Virology and Immunology at the Southwest Foundation for Biological Research, decided to pay a house call—on their homes.

What he found was not pretty. Large amounts of mold, bacteria, and other infectious nasties were floating in the air.

The cause? Dr. Jacobs traced the problem to contaminated central air-conditioning units. "These systems are often poorly designed," he says. "They should be inspected frequently, but often the homeowner has no access to the interior."

With the help of local heating and air-conditioning contractors, Dr. Jacobs opened up sealed access panels to reveal the problem.

"Until you've actually seen one of these heavily contaminated units, you have a hard time realizing just how bad it can be," he warns. Actual mushrooms have been found growing away in the warm moistness behind those sealed panels.

The slime and mold so often uncovered takes root when the system's drain to the outside becomes clogged.

"Most homeowners don't even realize that they have a drain going outside from their central air-conditioning system," explains Dr. Jacobs. "But every system has a drain, and if yours isn't dripping water when the system is on, you've probably got a problem."

If you keep cool with central air, Dr. Jacobs feels that it is definitely worth the time and trouble to create a way to keep an eye on your system.

If one look tells you that it's contaminated (with visible mold and slime), clean the area with a solution of 10 parts water to 1 part bleach. Never use bleach full strength. And never mix bleach with ammonia, warns Dr. Jacobs, or you'll wind up breathing in fumes toxic enough to be used in chemical warfare!

To keep the system clean, drop one of those swimming pool chlorine tablets into the drip pan once a month. And keep an eye on that drain.

The materials used in your system are also a factor, warn many experts. If the area involved is metal, the bleach solution should clean it up nicely. But if fiberglass or other porous materials have been invaded by mold and mildew, they may need to be replaced. Once deeply ingrained in such materials, mold is extremely difficult to remove.

Have your heating/air-conditioning contractor replace the contaminated portions with easily cleaned metal parts, and you'll be able to handle future maintenance yourself.

Ductwork Danger

Central forced-air heating and air-conditioning systems are designed for ease of climate control. But their actual physical design also makes them a powerful source of potential problems.

The ductwork that actually carries the warmed or cooled air to each room can act like potting soil for pathogens. Pounds of mold, bacteria, and fungus-infested dust are often uncovered in the neglected ductwork of a single home.

When the warm or cool air generated by the system blows down these unclean corridors, it carries those nasty microorganisms right to your nose. For people allergic to molds, the result can be a full-court press of allergic symptoms.

But unlike other allergens, such as pollen, a mold explosion can also affect the nonallergic—sometimes severely. Symptoms can include headaches, fatigue, sneezing, and nasal and eye problems. If the mold continues to flourish, the people in the home may even develop a serious pneumonia-like condition called hypersensitivity pneumonitis.

Visible dust or mold on the registers is a clue that your ductwork could use some work.

To check them, put on a face mask (available at any hardware store) and unscrew the grates covering the ductwork in several rooms. If there's a lot of nasty-looking stuff on the back of the registers or in the ducts themselves (look with a flashlight), contact a commercial duct-cleaning service and have those unwanted organisms evicted.

If you have just moved into a home or if you haven't had your ductwork cleaned in 10 to 12 years, you should definitely bring in professional cleaners.

In the meantime, you can temporarily reduce the misery by taping several layers of cheesecloth over the registers—especially in the bedrooms. But this will also cut the air flow and reduce heating and cooling efficiency and should only be used for a short period of time. Right after you seal up the last vent, call the cavalry to come clear out your dirty ducts.

Heating Problems

One expert doesn't think you should call autumn "the cold and flu season." He has renamed this time of year, when certain types of illness seem to flourish, "the furnace season."

When the heat comes on in homes, he explains, a lot of potential problems are activated that can foul the indoor air so badly you'll feel like you've got the flu.

A 1987 study on indoor air quality performed for the U.S. Department of Energy agrees. Although the causes of indoor air problems were found to vary widely from home to home, "combustion products" were a frequent culprit. Whenever there's combustion—a flame of any kind—it's going to consume precious oxygen and give off deadly ingredients that most of us simply cannot tolerate.

Carbon monoxide is the deadliest of those combustion products. And it taints indoor air frequently. Often misdiagnosed as a seasonal virus or flu, carbon monoxide exposure sickens untold numbers as it kills an estimated 3,800 people a year. Potential indoor sources include gas appliances, oil burners, wood stoves, and kerosene heaters.

Knowing its symptoms can save your life: 92 percent of people who are exposed to dangerous levels feel fatigued, and 85 percent have headaches that vanish after they've been away from their homes (or cars, if that's where the problem is) for a while.

Be warned—physicians admit that the problem is frustratingly difficult to diagnose in a doctor's office or hospital. People seeking medical attention are often told they have a cold or flu and are sent right back to the source of their problem.

The solution? There are several.

You should check all gas appliances (including water heaters) to make sure that the flame burns pure blue. If there's a trace of yellow or an irregular shape to the flame, call the gas company.

Never cook on a gas stove without using a fan or something else that actually vents the air to the outside.

Have your oil burner inspected every year, and check chimneys regularly to make sure that they're not blocked.

Kerosene heaters are especially unsafe. Have you ever known anyone to actually open a window in the room to provide the ventilation they require? Without that fresh air source, they quickly consume oxygen and replace it with a laundry list of potentially harmful gases.

Older models pollute the worst. If you have a newer, low-pollution model and you feel you have to use it, keep the wick at the indicated length. Too high a wick will cause smelly soot to foul the air; too low a wick will allow lots of carbon monoxide to invade your home.

And you must open a window if you want to be really safe. Better to bag the kerosene and choose almost any other kind of space heater. Anything short of an open fire on the living room floor would be an improvement.

Wood stoves? Researchers from the Indoor Environment Program of the University of California found that these much-maligned heaters don't produce a lot of indoor air pollution.

The exception, they note, is the old-style Franklin stove. This type, which has gaps and openings in its structure that allow smoke to escape, was found to really mangle the indoor air in real-life testing situations. Newer, airtight stoves were found to release only small amounts of pollutants into the indoor air—and then only during firing up and refueling. So limit the amount of time your firebox door is open, and you can enjoy that oh-so-comforting warmth without sacrificing indoor air quality.

If you have a garage that's attached to your home, never start the car until your garage doors are wide open, and turn the car off as soon as possible.

Indoor tune-ups are an especially bad idea. All car maintenance functions should be performed outside.

Tobacco smoke—one of the most common "combustion causes" of poor indoor air quality—is also the most preventable. An end to lighting up indoors often means the end of a lot of health complaints as well, say many experts.

Yes, cigarettes give off carbon monoxide (and smokers' blood generally shows high levels of the deadly gas when tested). But a complete list of all the chemicals, carcinogens, and pollutants released by burning cigarettes would fill this page—at least.

The Formaldehyde Fix

Many people became personally acquainted with the problems caused by indoor air pollution when formaldehyde foam was pumped into the walls of their homes as insulation.

The unstable formaldehyde didn't stay put. It "gassed out" into the air and irritated people's skin, eyes, and throat. It nauseated them and gave them headaches.

Soon many trailer homes were found to have alarmingly high levels of formaldehyde in their indoor air. The cause was felt to be lack of ventilation combined with heavy use of the kind of man-made materials that "off gas" the irritating chemical.

Formaldehyde can be present in a wide array of household items: High levels in homes are generally caused by new carpeting and other fabric furnishings, particleboard cabinets and other furniture, and even the very plywoods and glues used to build the home itself.

Luckily, experts say that use of the chemical is on the decline. Shop around, ask questions, don't be shy about calling manufacturers or local builders, and you should be able to find just about any product in a formaldehyde-free form.

For materials already in place, problems caused by high formaldhyde levels should always be on the decline. That's because the worst "off gassing" occurs during the first few months, and detectable indoor levels drop greatly after the first year.

You don't need fancy gadgets to detect high levels of formaldehyde, either—researchers assure us that a strong chemical smell generally accompanies problem levels.

You can also purge a lot of the chemical out of new materials quickly by exposing them to high temperatures and high humidity, explains Suresh Relwani, a research engineer who specializes in accurately measuring indoor formaldehyde levels. (Just don't stand around breathing the formaldehyde as it's leaving!)

For regular maintenance of your indoor air, the opposite is in order. Keeping the temperature and humidity as low as comfortably possible in your home will also keep formaldehyde emissions low.

Levels emitted by new materials could drop greatly if you "cook" the formaldehyde out with a few days of high temperature and high humidity (while you take advantage of a "getaway weekend" somewhere) and then keep them cool and dry afterward.

The Real Villain: OPEC!

The Arab oil embargo and subsequent energy crisis did more than teach us how to get stuff done while we wait in line for gas. It also inspired a generation to seal up every hole in their homes in the name of energy efficiency.

What researchers soon discovered, however, was that sealing out the cold air also sealed in stale air and pollutants. Many experts feel that the widespread problem of radon pollution in homes is greatly worsened by this air-tightness obsession.

Mark Swanson, of the Allergic Diseases Research Lab of the Mayo Clinic, found that concentrations of allergens and pollutants were 38 times higher in a superinsulated home than in a normal one. To see if an air cleaner would help, he put a high-efficiency HEPA filter on the furnace of a typical "tight" energy-efficient home. Even after eight months of HEPA filtering, the air in the energy-efficient house was still five times worse than in a normal "leaky" home.

Levels of pollutants that might go unnoticed in a normal "leaky" home can accumulate to cause "sick building syndrome" and its symptoms—including headaches, fatigue, and nausea—in a superinsulated home.

"Ventilation," explains Mark Schenker, M.D., director of

the Occupational and Environmental Health Unit for the University of California, is the solution to stale air problems. "Enough regular air changes per hour and the problem is completely solved," he explains.

So if you've caulked, insulated, and triple-glazed everything in sight, it might be time to let a little fresh air into your life.

A good energy-saving way to accomplish that is with an air-to-air heat exchanger. These devices trap heat from the exhausted stale air that they force out of the house and use it to warm the incoming fresh air. They recover about 75 percent of the energy that would normally be lost through conventional ventilation.

AIDS Update: What to Quit Worrying About

There's no question: The fear of AIDS is far more widespread than AIDS itself. There's plenty of evidence, though, that much of the fear is unnecessary. And harmful.

Our best protection against the fear—and the virus—is scientific knowledge. The knowledge boils down to this: It's tough to get the AIDS virus. It's tough, or impossible, even in situations where you might think AIDS would be inevitable.

In the interest of peace of mind, AIDS experts present 15 situations you've probably wondered about—and reveals why the odds are in your favor:

1. You can't get AIDS simply sharing an elevator with one—or even a dozen—AIDS patients. Unlike the common-cold virus, the AIDS virus infects blood cells—it can't become airborne in breath.

"The AIDS virus hijacks genes and enzymes from white blood cells to replicate itself," says AIDS expert Margaret A. Fischl, M.D., of the University of Miami. "It can't do that outside the body."

2. You can't get AIDS simply sharing a Perrier or pizza with someone who's infected. The infected person could leave saliva on your Perrier and pizza, and you'd still be safe, for two reasons: First, the virus is rarely found in saliva. In a study of 83 AIDS patients, for instance, the virus turned up in the saliva of only 1 (*New England Journal of Medicine*).

Second, saliva inactivates the virus. In studies of households and families with an infected member, AIDS patients shared food and drink, plates, glasses, cutlery, and toothbrushes with uninfected people. No one got AIDS this way (*New England Journal of Medicine*).

3. You can't get AIDS by simply shaking hands with or hugging an infected person. The virus isn't found in sweat or on skin. In the household studies, people hugged and had lots of other close, nonsexual contact. Not one case of AIDS was spread this way (*New England Journal of Medicine*).

"The virus has to get into the bloodstream to infect cells," Dr. Fischl says. "That doesn't happen when you shake someone's hand or hug them."

4. You can't get AIDS simply by being sneezed on or coughed on by an AIDS patient. The AIDS virus has not been found in the phlegm or nasal mucus of infected people. Experts, including the U.S. Surgeon General, agree there's no evidence that the virus spreads through this kind of casual contact.

5. You can't get AIDS by simply sitting on a toilet seat, even if the person who used it before you was infected. "The virus can't live on a toilet seat," says Charles P. Fallis of the Centers for Disease Control. "It dies immediately in open air."

The virus has sometimes been found in urine, but in quantities so small scientists think the virus isn't transmitted this way. The AIDS virus has also been isolated in feces. But in 11 studies of more than 700 AIDS patients who lived and shared toilets with uninfected people, the virus never spread this way. In no known case has contact with urine or feces—on a toilet seat or anyplace else—led to infection (*Journal of the American Medical Association*).

6. You can't get AIDS by simply swimming in a pool or soaking in a hot tub, even if someone else in the water is infected. "Since there's no evidence of infection through much more intensive exposures to urine, the risk from urine in swimming pools and hot tubs is negligible," says Alan R. Lifson, M.D., of the San Francisco Department of Public Health's AIDS office. And, as stated previously, the virus isn't found in sweat or on skin, and the risk from feces is negligible. Anyway, the virus can't survive in water.

7. You can't get AIDS by simply kissing an infected person on the cheek or lips. Again, there's no evidence saliva transmits the virus. People in the household studies kissed each other without spreading AIDS.

Still, the Surgeon General advises against French kissing someone who might be infected. Transmission through French kissing has never been documented. But since the virus has been isolated in saliva (although in rare cases), it's sensible to play it safe.

"Even in more intimate settings, there have been no documented cases of transmission by saliva," says Dr. Lifson. "Therefore, the risk of infection from kissing on the cheek or lips is negligible."

8. You can't get AIDS by simply eating in a restaurant, even if the chef is infected. It's already established that you can't get AIDS through contact with saliva, sweat, and skin. But what if—in a worst-case scenario—an infected chef cuts himself and bleeds on a salad that you later have with your dinner? The risk is still negligible. Experts say that the amount of virus that could be present in a few drops of infected blood is scant. And the likelihood that the virus could survive passage through the digestive tract is extremely small.

9. You can't get AIDS by simply donating blood. The myth that the virus could be acquired this way started because of the risk of receiving infected blood. People twisted the concept around and figured it's risky to give blood. But it's just not true, according to the Centers for Disease Control. There's no risk whatsoever when needles are used only once, as they are for blood donors in the United States.

The AIDS virus may spread on unsterilized needles during acupuncture, tattooing, and ear piercing. Sterilization, however, eliminates all risks. Dipping needles in a 1-to-10 dilution of bleach, alcohol, hydrogen peroxide, or Lysol kills the virus. So does 10 minutes of 140°F heat.

10. You can't get AIDS by being bitten by mosquitoes or other insects. This myth gained currency when researchers theorized that mosquitoes might have spread AIDS in Belle Glade, Florida, where an outbreak occurred from 1982 to 1987 among people with no known risk factors.

The myth—and the Belle Glade scare—was laid to rest by three pieces of evidence. First, AIDS is age-specific. Most infected people are aged 20 to 49. Insects don't discriminate by age; sexually transmitted diseases do. Second, in Belle Glade, scientists eventually found sex and intravenous drug abuse were the routes of infection. Third, there's no evidence of the AIDS virus in insects (*Science*).

11. You can't get AIDS from the hepatitis-B vaccine or gamma-globulin shot (used to prevent hepatitis A). This myth started because the gamma-globulin shot and one form of the hepatitis-B vaccine are derived from blood, raising the possibility of the AIDS virus being present in thses products.

But despite administration of these preventives to thousands of people, no cases of AIDS have been linked to the vaccine or gamma-globulin shot. The process used to make them inactivates all known viruses, including the AIDS virus.

12. You can't get AIDS from pets and other nonhuman animals, even those infected with AIDS-like diseases. The AIDS virus grows in chimpanzees, gibbons, and rabbits. A similar virus grows in baboons, macaques, and the African green monkey. "But unless you inject yourself with their blood, the chance of infection from these animals is negligible," says Thomas J. Kindt, Ph.D., of the National Institute of Allergy and Infectious Diseases.

Feline leukemia and certain diseases of goats and horses are, like AIDS, immunodeficiency diseases. "But none of these viruses can grow in human cells," Dr. Kindt says.

13. You can't get AIDS by simply working or going to school with someone who has AIDS. No case of AIDS is known or suspected to have been spread by children in schools or day-care centers.

But what if blood from an infected child somehow comes in contact with an uninfected child's open wound? Infection is still highly unlikely. Scientists know this from doctors and nurses accidentally exposed to the virus.

THE THREE KNOWN WAYS YOU CAN GET AIDS

1. You can get AIDS through sexual contact with an infected person. This is the most common way AIDS spreads. Your most important precaution: Don't choose a sex partner at high risk for AIDS. Monogamy and condoms also reduce risk.

The Centers for Disease Control (CDC) report close to 47,000 AIDS cases among homosexual or bisexual men and about 3,200 cases among heterosexuals.

2. You can get AIDS through infected organ or tissue transplants and inoculation or infusion with infected blood. Most people who received blood since April 1985, when blood screening was introduced, are at low risk. With screening, the risk from blood transfusions has been minimized. Scientists estimate the risk of infection from one transfusion is now between 1 in 100,000 and 1 in 1 million.

The virus has been transmitted through kidney, heart, liver, pancreas, and bone transplants, but only in 28 reported cases worldwide, according to the CDC.

Contaminated needles, often shared by drug abusers, also spread the virus. About 14,800 IV drug abusers are known to have been infected.

3. Infants can get AIDS from infected mothers. Mothers can transmit the virus to infants across the placenta or during delivery. In one case, infection probably spread through breast milk. More than 900 children born to high-risk parents have been reported infected.

Even with direct inoculation—doctors and nurses accidentally sticking themselves with an infected needle—the AIDS virus seldom follows. One estimate puts the chance of infection from such a direct-inoculation accident at 1 in 286 (*New England Journal of Medicine*).

The household studies show the safety of casual contact among adults. No household members, except children born to infected mothers, sexual partners of patients, or people with other risks, got the virus. No evidence, anywhere in the world, shows casual transmission of AIDS at school or work.

14. You can't get AIDS by simply visiting an infected person's home. After all the other evidence we've mentioned, this should be obvious. But it isn't to everyone. At least 11 household studies show that there's no risk whatsoever from living with an AIDS patient—even for long periods of time— let alone visiting one (*American Journal of Epidemiology*).

15. You can't get AIDS by having sex with someone who isn't infected. Really, you can't.

Groups at highest risk include homosexual and bisexual men and intravenous drug abusers from big cities; hemophili-

---

SEX SAFETY:
THE TRUE RISKS OF GETTING AIDS

The risk of acquiring the AIDS virus from one episode of penis/vagina intercourse with someone of unknown AIDS status who *isn't* in a high-risk group is 1 in 50 million (with condom) or 1 in 5 million (without).

The risk of acquiring the AIDS virus from one episode of penis/vagina intercourse with someone of unknown AIDS status who *is* in a high-risk group is 1 in 100,000 to 1 in 10,000 (with condom) or 1 in 10,000 to 1 in 1,000 (without). These odds vary because of differing rates of infection among high-risk groups.

The risk of acquiring the AIDS virus from one episode of penis/vagina intercourse with someone who has tested negative for AIDS but continues to engage in high-risk behavior (needle-sharing or sexual intercourse with a member of a high-risk group) is 1 in 500,000 (with condom) or 1 in 50,000 (without).

The risk of acquiring the AIDS virus from one episode of penis/vagina intercourse with someone who has tested positive for AIDS is 1 in 5,000 (with condom) or 1 in 500 (without).

With one exception—anal intercourse—other kinds of sexual activities carry much less risk.

The above odds worsen with repeated heterosexual intercourse. After 500 times with someone who tests positive and doesn't use a condom, for example, the chance of being infected is two in three.

acs; female prostitutes; heterosexuals from Haiti and central Africa where AIDS is common; and recipients of multiple blood transfusions from areas where AIDS was common between 1983 and 1985.

Despite what you may have heard, the AIDS virus is relatively hard to get sexually (see "Sex Safety: The True Risks of Getting AIDS"). Part of the reason is that the virus isn't easily transmitted in a single or few exposures.

Bouncing Back from a Stay in the Hospital

Postoperative recovery is a long process, usually taking upward of two months. That's two months of lying on your back, two months of seeing whatever strides you made toward fitness prior to your hospital stay go down the drain.

"The biggest mistake people make after having an operation or being laid up in the hospital for a while is that they try to start where they left off," says Phil Dunphy, an exercise physiologist and physical therapist at HEAR (Health through Exercise and Rehabilitation) in Red Bank, New Jersey. "Studies show that if you work out for seven weeks and then don't work out for another seven, you're back in the condition you were in when you started—probably even worse."

And while the road to optimum fitness is a long one—especially after a months-long layoff—it can be reached by taking it one step at a time with walking.

Whether you're recovering from a heart attack, surgery, or pregnancy and delivery, walking is the "perfect" exercise for the comeback trail, say experts. It's also the ideal workout for those suffering from arthritis or other degenerative diseases that make other forms of exercise painful.

"Walking is the perfect choice for recovering patients because it gives them what they want: a general improvement in body tone, in aerobic health, and in overall body function, without stressing the body too much," says D. W. Edington, Ph.D., director of the University of Michigan Fitness Research Center. "Most of the time, recovering from surgery, a heart attack, or a pregnancy is a four- to eight-week process; it takes that long for the body to recover, and it should be a gradual process. Walking is ideal for that."

Adds Dunphy: "Before you start walking, it's important to start a good flexibility program. You should start slowly and work up toward stretching for about 20 minutes a day. It doesn't have to be anything heavy-duty; sitting in a chair and doing leg lifts is fine."

When you hit the road, Robert Goldszer, M.D., a blood pressure specialist and assistant professor of medicine at Harvard Medical School, recommends that most recovering heart patients strive toward gentle walking for 20-minute stretches, three to five times weekly. "Of course, the most important thing to do first is check with your doctor," he adds. "When recovering from a heart attack, it's very important to be closely monitored when doing exercise. That means learning how to check your pulse." Normally, exercisers are attempting to work toward maintaining between 60 and 85 percent of their maximum heart rate zone. But after a hospital stay, you should probably not exceed 40 percent. As strength increases, workouts can, too.

Besides walking, Dunphy, Dr. Edington, and Dr. Goldszer also recommend gentle bicycling and swimming for recovering patients.

What to Avoid

Some types of exercise, however, should be avoided after a hospital stay, especially by recovering heart patients. Weight lifting, isometrics, and other resistance exercises can be too taxing on your body—and usually require holding your breath, which can result in elevated blood pressure and cause undue strain on the heart.

Women recovering from pregnancy—especially those who have undergone a cesarean delivery—should also avoid exercises that work the abdominal muscles, such as sit-ups (although women who've had a vaginal delivery may do sit-ups under the direction of their physician). "Kegel exercises, which tighten the pelvic muscles, are excellent—both during pregnancy and following delivery," adds Dunphy.

High-impact aerobics, as well as any sport that requires a lot of jumping (such as basketball, volleyball, and running), should also be avoided by anyone recovering from heart attack, pregnancy, or surgery. And obviously, without first getting an okay from your doctor or physical therapist, avoid exercises that directly work any portion of your body that was operated on—for example, sit-ups for those who have had a hernia operation.

"The key to any recovery program is to realize that it's going to take time and not to expect overnight miracles," says Dr. Edington. "Realize that a tremendous insult has been done to your body and it takes time to recover. But once you start an exercise program—and stick with it—you can be in better shape than you ever were before."

The Ins and Outs of Insomnia

Poor Socrates. Seems he was an insomniac who spent all night philosophizing while his wife was trying to sleep. One night, while he was expressing his views on the nature of the universe, she did likewise on the nature of his sleeping habits—by dumping on his head the contents of their bedroom chamber pot, the ancient Greeks' version of a toilet. That, no doubt, led to further philosophic discussion.

You can go months without food and years without sex, but miss a few nights of shut-eye and you feel something like Socrates' shampoo. But as known by the nation's 120 million insomniacs—many of them hard-driving achievers who take their work home and into bed—lack of sleep doesn't necessarily mean lack of performance.

"We all need sleep, but we all don't need the same amount," says Ernest Hartmann, M.D., a sleep researcher for

25 years and director of two sleep-disorder centers in Boston. "A lot depends on your personality and what kind of life you lead." People who get along on less sleep tend to be very busy people who are happy with their lives.

Whether or not they're happy, executives tend to get less sleep—not always by choice. In fact, they even have their own brand of executive insomnia, one of the 120 sleep disorders recognized by the Association of Sleep Disorders Centers in Rochester, Minnesota. Called fibrositis, it is common among intense perfectionists, especially women between 25 and 50, who suffer from shallow sleep because the wake center of their brain remains active.

Factors besides work have an effect on the quality and quantity of our sleep. Men seem to sleep more deeply than women, says Elliott R. Phillips, M.D., medical director of the North Valley Sleep Disorders Center near Los Angeles.

Age also plays a role: As time goes by, we need less sleep. Newborns and infants sleep about 16 hours a day—spending almost half the time dreaming. As we reach senior citizenship, the standard drops to 6 hours, with less than 2 of them spent in dreamland. The turning point seems to occur around age 50, when sleep cycles change, resulting in more middle-of-the-night awakenings, shorter dreams, and less overall sleep.

The Good News about Bad Sleep

Aside from seeing too many late-night B movies, there's little harm from getting too few ZZZ's, researchers say. "You cannot die of sleep deprivation," says Dr. Hartmann, one of the country's leading sleep researchers. "If you go three or four days without sleep, you'll feel awful, but it affects your performance less than you think."

Translation: Don't worry if you miss a night or two of sleep—even before a job interview or other important event. The body adapts to short-term sleep deprivation and makes up for lost sleep on another night. In fact, says Peter Hauri, Ph.D., director of the Insomnia Program at the sleep-disorder center at the Mayo Clinic, "It's probably better that we tend to lose sleep on nights before important days. Your adrenaline keeps you going the next day and makes up for the lost sleep."

Lack of sleep seems to affect us more psychologically than physically. "An acute lack of sleep doesn't affect your physical performance, but it does affect your attitude," says Daniel Wagner, M.D., of the Sleep-Wake Disorders Center at Cornell University Medical Center. "Not getting enough sleep induces a kind of pessimism. Outside observers probably wouldn't notice this, but you would. You tend to be more critical of yourself when you don't sleep enough."

But chronic sleep deprivation takes its toll. When an American disc jockey went without sleep for more than 200

TIPS FOR BETTER SLEEP

For better shut-eye, shut off caffeine, alcohol, and nicotine close to lights-out. Sleeping pills are also a no-no; they lose their effectiveness within a few days.

Physical activity at night can keep your body revving come slumbertime. For sleeping's sake, the best time to exercise is late afternoon or early evening.

Doing activities in bed other than sleeping doesn't help either. "All too many insomniacs read or watch television in bed, and it keeps them awake," says Daniel Wagner, M.D., of the Sleep-Wake Disorders Center at Cornell University Medical Center. "If you have trouble sleeping, my advice is to eliminate almost all waking activities from bed, if not the bedroom itself."

That can mean *all* bedroom activities. While sex can be the best (or at least most fun) sleeping pill around, those anxious about their sex lives are urged not to participate just prior to sleep time. "Otherwise, you'll be up all night worrying about it," says one sleep researcher.

Anxiety—whether about sex or other matters—is another sleep buster. "Don't do your checkbook and then jump into bed," says Dr. Wagner. "You need time to unwind, to clear your mind. You need to do something to take your mind off your worries."

And that includes worries about sleep. "The biggest mistake people make is trying to make sleep happen," he says. "You can't make sleep happen. You'll make it up when you need to."

hours—or more than eight days—he reported hallucinations and paranoia. Sleep researchers now believe that the hallucinations he reported were actually dreams he experienced. "When you're deprived of sleep, there comes a point where the body will make sure it gets some," says Dr. Phillips. "You *will* sleep and experience dreams, though you may not know it."

Napping: A Mixed Blessing

But how we get it depends on our individual body clock—and culture. "Everyone needs about 6 hours of sleep, but you don't have to get it all at once," says Dr. Hartmann. "A quarter of the world breaks up sleep into two segments—an afternoon siesta for a couple of hours and the rest at night."

Napping, though, can be mixed blessing. Since the first 90 minutes of sleep are the most refreshing and regenerative, a daytime nap may reduce stress (a common reason for insomnia) and result in a quick pick-me-up. One study even indicated that a daily 30-minute snooze may have contributed to a 30 percent decrease in incidence of heart attack among men. But too much napping can lead to sleeping disorders, especially in older men.

"Sleep disorders increase with age, and one reason is because the elderly tend to nap more frequently," says Michael Stevenson, Ph.D., director of the Insomnia Clinic at North Valley Sleep Disorder Center in Mission Hills, California. "When you get older, you tend to nap—and that keeps you up at night."

Unless you nap to catch up on lost sleep, that quick 40 winks can yield diminishing returns—doing the job usually reserved for our nightlife. "Your system operates on a narrow ability to synchronize with a 24-hour day," says Dr. Wagner. "Sleeping on a variable schedule can produce a situation like jet lag, even though you haven't physically moved out of your time zone. Your internal clock protests in two ways: It doesn't let you get to sleep as quickly, and it disrupts your sleep once sleep has started."

PILLOW TALK

Your sleeping position says a lot about your personality, say sleep researchers. For instance:

- Prong sleepers—the 25 percent who sleep on their stomach—are fussy and domineering "control" freaks who do not like the unexpected and try to avoid it whenever possible.
- Royal sleepers, who sleep on their backs. are self-reliant and assured, sometimes egoholics. This 7.5 percent of nighttime lumberjacks were usually favorite children or the center of attention. Many actors are said to sleep in this position, perhaps because it's the easiest way to bow in your sleep.
- Full-fetal sleepers spend their sack time on their sides, usually clutching an object to themselves in a tightly closed bud or ball. This 7.5 percent is said to be insecure and inhibited, and their position—usually guarding the midsection—indicates a strong desire for protection. Full-fetal sleepers tend to lie on the corners of the bed, usually facing outward.
- Semifetal sleepers—those who sleep on their sides, with open or exposed arms—are the most common. Representing 60 percent of the population, semifetals tend to be well-balanced and secure people with good common sense. In fact, semifetal is called the "good common sense" position because is allows you to conserve body heat without closing off air circulation around the body (like the full-fetal position). Right-handed semifetals tend to sleep on their right side, and vice versa.

His advice: Retire and awaken at the same time *every* day. If you get 2 hours of sleep during a daytime nap, expect to have 2 hours less sleep that night. Dr. Wagner says this also applies to sleeping late on weekends. "If you sleep late on weekends, it'll affect your next week's sleep."

How to Ask Smokers "Not to"—Nicely

Nonsmokers have fought for unfouled air with "Please don't smoke" signs, portable electric fans, and icy stares. But now it's serious. Now it's time to bring out the Ultimate Weapon—nonsmokers' etiquette. It's the art of polite ploys that help you get your fair share of smokeless air without embarrassing anyone or ruffling feathers—at work, at home, in restaurants, anywhere. To help you learn the fine points, here's Miss Etiquette, the intrepid (albeit imaginary) expert who answers some tough (but hypothetical) letters regarding the real (very real) problems that arise when smokers and nonsmokers mix.

Dear Miss Etiquette:
It's important to me to be proper. But the brouhaha over smoking has me confused. Isn't it courteous to let everyone do as he or she wishes?

Mixed Up in Peoria

Dear Mixed Up:
Wake up and smell the fresh air! Your sense of courtesy is passe. Today we know that cigarette smoking is not simply rude, but unhealthy. The new rule to write into your etiquette book is this: "The choice to smoke cannot interfere with the nonsmoker's right to breathe air free of tobacco smoke." This principle comes from none other than the U.S. Surgeon General.

For good reason. Evidence now indicates that passive, or involuntary, smokers—nonsmoking people who regularly breathe other people's smoke—run an increased risk for disease, including lung cancer. Cigarette smoke also irritates eyes, nose, and throat. Worst of all, as was pointed out in the 1986 Surgeon General's report, *The Health Consequences of Involuntary Smoking,* the children of parents who smoke suffer more respiratory problems and impaired lung growth than children of nonsmokers.

Dear Miss Etiquette:

I dine in restaurants frequently and often find myself seated near smokers. But I find it awkward to ask them not to smoke, so sometimes I just wave the smoke away with my hands and cough. But they don't get the hint. Is there a better way to handle this?

Reluctant to Speak

Dear Reluctant:

Since you're nervous about confronting smokers, it may be best for you to try to avoid the situation entirely. And that's getting easier to do. More and more restaurants offer no-smoking areas (in many states and cities, they're required by law), and some restaurants have banned smoking entirely. Local nonsmokers' groups may be able to steer you to them. You can also simply call ahead to inquire about a restaurant's arrangements for nonsmokers. If the manager tells you there are no separate accommodations, you can tell him or her that you'll refrain from visiting until there are.

Whether there's a nonsmoking section or not, always ask for seating away from the smokers as soon as you arrive at the restaurant. Another tip: Dine early, because the smoke gets thicker as the night wears on.

Let's say you've taken these precautions, and a smoker lights up nearby anyway. Your typical response—coughing, waving your hands, maybe grumbling—is called "passive-aggressive behavior." And it's the worst possible course, says psychologist Barry Lubetkin, Ph.D., director of the Institute for Behavior Therapy in New York City. "People have the most resistance to change when others aren't completely frank with them. If someone waves away the smoke but doesn't say anything to the smoker, it gives the smoker a chance to disengage himself from responsibility for his act.

"But if you confront the smoker politely, he must take responsibility for what he's doing. And if you can provide him with an alternative that saves face, it generally works."

Dr. Lubetkin suggests that you try one of these lines.

"I would appreciate it if you blew your smoke in another direction."

"I understand that you want to continue smoking, and that's fine, but could you hold your cigarette in your other hand?"

"We'll be leaving in 10 minutes. If you can hold off smoking until then, we'd appreciate it."

If these don't work, "escalate" your request, says Dr. Lubetkin.

"Would you mind putting out your cigarette? This is a no-smoking area."

"Excuse me, I'm allergic to cigarette smoke (or I have trouble breathing cigarette smoke), and I must ask you to put out your cigarette."

Virtually all smokers will comply to these last two lines, says Dr. Lubetkin. If they don't, escalate a little more by asking your waiter or waitress to make the request. In the rare cases where all requests fail, ask to be moved to another table.

When you're bothered by smoke at a restaurant, do mention it to the waiter or the manager, or write a note on your check. "If patrons don't say anything, restaurateurs think there is no demand for nonsmoking sections," says Regina Carlson, executive director of New Jersey GASP (Group against Smoking Pollution). "But I think people are afraid to speak up."

Dear Miss Etiquette:
What on earth do I do when my smoking in-laws attend a party I'm throwing? I don't want to alienate them or my nonsmoking guests, and I don't want my house smelling like tobacco afterward.

Frantic at the Thought

Dear Frantic:
Here are some approaches to try.

When you telephone smokers with an invitation, say warmly, "We are so eager to see you; I hope you can attend. You should know, however, that this will be a no-smoking party." You could also say, "We are expecting several guests who, like us, have trouble tolerating cigarette smoke."

Put a no-smoking sign on the door or in the entry hall. New

Jersey GASP offers members a sign that says, "Welcome to another smoke-free home." Remove all ashtrays so you're not sending mixed messages.

If you wish, offer an area where guests can smoke— ideally, outdoors, on a patio or well-ventilated porch. For winter affairs, you may wish to allow guests to smoke by the fireplace (if there's a fire) or in a bathroom (with the exhaust fan going).

Miss Etiquette does not wish to rush you into motherhood, but if you do produce grandchildren for your in-laws, it will be easier to express your wishes to them. Simply remind them that children's health can be harmed by secondhand smoke: "We want your grandchildren's air to be clean and healthy, and I'm sure you agree that smoky air would be bad for them to breathe."

Dear Miss Etiquette:
It's one thing to prevent guests from smoking in your home, but what if your spouse is polluting the indoor air? I love my wife very much, but I hate her pack-a-day habit. I've begged and pleaded, but nothing helps. Can you?

At Wits' End

Dear Wits:
Nagging is not only impolite, it's ineffective—it only makes the smoker more obstinate. The first thing you should do to reduce household strife and protect yourself and your children is negotiate on a smoking zone. "Find a place that's not a common area, ideally outdoors," says Joan Belson, R.N., a smoking-cessation counselor in Newton, Massachusetts. "If the smoker agrees to smoke only there, you agree to not nag anymore."

If your wife must smoke indoors, choose a well-ventilated room and keep the door shut. That will reduce, but not eliminate, the indoor pollution.

None of this, of course, changes the fact that you want your spouse to quit. But you can't make that decision for her, and as you've noticed, pestering doesn't help. "I think you need to respect an addiction," says Belson, herself an ex-smoker. "Don't make quitting a condition of love."

But in a loving way, you can help your spouse find incentives to quit. "We've found that people quit according to very particular idiosyncratic needs," says Dr. Lubetkin. He recalls a patient who couldn't break the tobacco habit until the night his young daughter said to him, "Daddy, I don't want to kiss you anymore because your breath smells." That did it.

Enrolling a smoker in a quitting program against his or her wishes isn't a wise investment. But you can hand them literature on free or low-cost, self-guided quitting programs, such as the American Lung Association's "Freedom from Smoking in 20 Days." About 20 percent of people who try "minimal intervention" programs like this quit successfully, says psychologist Lois Biener, Ph.D., director of the Worksite Smoking Program at the Miriam Hospital in Providence, Rhode Island.

When your spouse does decide to quit, that's when your attitude can definitely make a big difference. "Research indicates that people who are successful at quitting report that their spouses or the people they lived with gave them positive forms of support," says Dr. Biener. "They helped them think about other things to do when they wanted a cigarette, took them to a movie, gave them rewards, or praised them for not smoking."

Dear Miss Etiquette:
I work in an office full of smokers. Even my boss smokes! I'm afraid that it's making me sick, but I don't know how to talk to them about it without triggering anger (mine and theirs)— and maybe getting fired. What can I do?

Employed but Wheezing

Dear Employed:
You're in a very difficult situation, but the fresh winds of change are blowing your way. Robert Rosner, executive director of the Smoking Policy Institute in Seattle, Washington, estimates that half of all U.S. workplaces have nonsmoking policies—and the number is growing every day. Some nonsmoking rules are mandated by local or state law.

Where should you begin to change policy in your own workplace? Where you shouldn't start is with sarcasm or anger. "This is an emotional issue that you want to turn into a business issue," says Rosner. "The nonsmoker has to be very professional and has to present a factual business case for looking into the issue."

So start by educating yourself about the health effects of smoke on nonsmokers. Then you can do something as simple as put a note in a suggestion box. If you work for a large company, contact the department that handles employee relations, or health and safety. Get other nonsmokers to express their concerns about their own health, too.

When you do bring your case to the top, says Rosner, don't declare that you want a total ban on smoking. "It's much more effective to push for a review of the issue. Say, 'I believe we have a problem. I would like to explore it; do I have your permission?' It's also less threatening."

Then you or your colleagues may have to do a little more research to begin putting together your "business case" for a work-site nonsmoking policy. It should include information about

- The economic costs of smoking to employers. The extra cost to an employer of a smoking employee can run to $5,000 annually, including higher costs for absenteeism, insurance, and office cleaning, according to the Smoking Policy Institute.
- The possibility of employee lawsuits. More and more non-smokers are winning lawsuits against their employers as a result of suffering from exposure to smoke. Nonsmokers don't always win, but those with medical complaints, such as smoke allergies or cardiovascular or respiratory problems, have the best chance in court.
- Success stories of companies that have restricted smoking.

Fortunately, there are many organizations that can help you gather and present this material. The Smoking Policy Institute, for example, can send you a packet of information and offers a persuasive video on workplace smoking to show to employers and employees.

If your company absolutely refuses to do anything about secondhand smoke, then one option is to consult a lawyer. In some states, you can receive unemployment compensation while pursuing this kind of lawsuit. Sometimes, when bosses realize they can be sued, their attitudes change. You can say, "I've overheard people talking about lawsuits"—but don't mention you're the one talking about them.

The easiest way to find out about the laws in your area is to contact your local nonsmoking organization or American Lung Association. You can ask them about proposed legislation, too, in case you want to lobby your lawmakers for changes in the law that can help everyone breathe easier.

Cholesterol Q & A

Cholesterol misinformation abounds. Confusion is rampant. Every day, it seems, there's a new study—contradicting the last one. To bring order to this chaos, a distinguished panel of cholesterol experts gives the fat facts—straight.

They give some good news about cookies, crackers, peanut butter, beans, oat bran, and fish. They give not-so-good news about "no cholesterol" foods. And they give lots of advice to reduce cholesterol and heart risks.

All this and more from the nation's top cholesterol-busters: James W. Anderson, M.D.; Andrea Bonanome, M.D.; the husband-and-wife team of William E. Connor, M.D., and Sonja L. Connor; and Kenneth H. Cooper, M.D. Check their advice. Then check any confusion at the door.

Which has the potential to raise cholesterol more, a 12-ounce T-bone steak or a three-egg omelet?

That's easy: the omelet—but not just because of its choking (745 milligrams) dose of cholesterol. What gives the omelet its heart-attacking edge is its combined cholesterol and saturated-fat content.

Yes, eating cholesterol raises blood cholesterol. But eating saturated fat seems to raise blood cholesterol still more, shutting down receptors in the liver that normally suck cholesterol from blood.

Although the T-bone has less cholesterol than the omelet, it shouldn't be a staple, either. Sonja Connor reckons the

T-bone steak totals a full-day's ration of these two artery pluggers.

Do labels stating "100% vegetable oil" or "no cholesterol" guarantee heart-healthy food?

No. And, worse, they can be very misleading.

First, keep in mind that only animal fats contain cholesterol. Plants do not. So, it's redundant to label a product both "100% vegetable oil" and "no cholesterol." Most manufacturers do so to underscore the product's health value. But those labels can be misleading. They imply the product is perfectly suited to a heart-healthy diet. In truth, some "no cholesterol" and "100% vegetable oil" foods contain a lot of saturated fat. Coconut and palm oil, for instance, are highly saturated.

"Hydrogenated," a word among the ingredients of cookies and crackers, means "saturated." In moderation, though, low-fat cookies and crackers are okay. The Connors, for instance, eat gingersnaps and low-fat crackers.

Moderation is key to another often-hydrogenated "no cholesterol" food, peanut butter. When you make a sandwich, go easy on the peanut butter—it's half fat. But peanut butter beats a cheese sandwich or hamburger, says Dr. Connor. Hamburger and most cheeses are high in saturated fat and cholesterol.

If saturated fat and cholesterol are the culprits in our diet, why does the American Heart Association recommend that we limit our intake of all fats to under 30 percent of our total calories?

First, because no fat is 100 percent unsaturated—or 100 percent saturated, for that matter. All fats are mixtures of saturated and unsaturated. Monounsaturated olive oil and polyunsaturated corn oil, for instance, are about 8 percent saturated. By cutting all fats across the board, then, you naturally reduce your intake of saturated fat.

Second, if you don't burn the calories, any fat makes you fat. Butter, for instance, has 102 calories per tablespoon. Olive oil has 119, and in excess, makes thighs thunder.

What's more, fat makes you fatter than other foods. Your body burns fewer calories storing fat than it does converting and storing carbohydrates.

Being overweight itself raises blood triglycerides. Like cholesterol, triglycerides burden the heart by obstructing arteries. (High triglyceride levels have been linked to heart attacks, especially in women.) The more you eat, the more triglycerides pour into your system. And as you put on excess weight, your liver is stimulated to produce more of its own triglycerides.

The bottom line: These experts back the American Heart Association's recommendations—and then some. Cut all fat to 20 to 25 percent of calories, say Dr. Anderson and Dr. Connor. People with dangerously high cholesterol should cut to 15 percent, Dr. Cooper says.

Where does research stand on Omega-3s?

It's unclear whether omega-3 fatty acids—found especially in mackerel, tuna, salmon, sardines, herring, pompano, trout, and other fish—reduce blood cholesterol, as early studies suggested. But they may reduce heart risks anyway.

First, they lower the liver's production of triglycerides. Second, they prevent clotting. Large amounts of fish oil alter the stickiness of blood platelets, making them less likely to clump together. When arteries are narrowed due to plaque deposits, a blood clot at the wrong place could cause a heart attack.

A third reason to eat fish: It's a lean alternative to beef. Three ounces of cooked Atlantic salmon (which is among the fattiest fish) contains only 5.4 grams of fat, compared to 17.5 grams of fat in 3 ounces of broiled rib-eye steak. Suffice it to say, the Connors eat fish three or four times a week.

Aside from eating fish and cutting cholesterol and fat, what other dietary steps lower blood cholesterol?

Reducing total calories and increasing soluble fiber (the kind that dissolves in water) lowers cholesterol, experts say. Soluble fiber—especially oat bran and beans, such as pinto or navy beans—flushes cholesterol from your body. (Insoluble fiber—the kind in wheat bran—does not have much effect on cholesterol.)

Dr. Anderson recommends about 6 grams of soluble fiber per day for most people. You can get that from ½ cup of oat bran cereal or 1 cup of beans. For people who can't reduce cholesterol with food alone, Dr. Anderson recommends psyllium, Metamucil's moving force. In his study, a teaspoon three times a day for eight weeks lowered cholesterol 15 percent.

Incidentally, the B vitamin niacin can also lower cholesterol. But the doses necessary to bring about such an effect are so high, it's considered a "drug" and should be used only under a doctor's supervision.

A middle-aged man with a stressful job downs eight cups of coffee and three alcoholic drinks a day. He has a potbelly and seldom exercises. What are his biggest heart risks? And what are the first and most important steps he should take to improve them?

His biggest risks, his potbelly and lack of exercise, go hand-in-hand—or hand-in-mouth. Alcohol, coffee, and stress may aggravate things. Even his age and sex are risks: Women have far fewer heart attacks until after menopause.

None of our experts recommends a sex change. But they disagree on what this potbellied man should do first. The Connors favor shifting his diet from fatty foods to low-fat dairy products, casseroles, fish, skinless poultry, beans, rice, pasta, fruits, and vegetables. That's not all. They want him to dry out to, at most, two alcoholic drinks three nights a week and three cups of coffee a day.

Dr. Cooper differs. "If I tell that man, 'You've got to stop drinking, lose weight and start exercising,' I'll never see him again. I'll just discourage him. That's why I usually work with exercise."

Dr. Cooper would start with walking 2 miles before dinner three times a week. Exercise, he says, raises HDL (high-density lipoprotein, the "good" cholesterol) and reduces triglycerides, appetite, stress and, sometimes, boozing. "With walking, he loses weight. He feels better and this augments the other things."

But even a slim 5-mile-a-day runner who shuns red meat can have clogged arteries. Why?

There are no sure things in the race against heart disease. It killed 52-year-old fitness guru Jim Fixx—after a run. In spite of his marathoner's body, Fixx's cholesterol was dangerously high. He also had a family history of heart disease: His father had a heart attack at 36 and died at 43.

Some people inherit a tendency to develop high cholesterol—and sometimes diets don't lower it enough. These people are "hyperresponders." Their livers produce excess cholesterol even when their diet is "low cholesterol." When their diet is bad, their liver goes into cholesterol overdrive. For them, drug therapy and close medical supervision—and a low-fat diet—may be the answer.

If you have a family history of heart disease, consult with a doctor.

How reliable are cholesterol tests?

Even $5 shopping-mall tests are generally reliable, although results can vary by 10 percent. "If someone has a cholesterol of 300, it could test 270 or 330," says Dr. Anderson. "But any of those is too high."

You can make your test more accurate. To get the best cholesterol measurement, fast and avoid vigorous exercise for 12 to 14 hours beforehand. But even if you've just exercised or eaten, get tested when you have a chance. At least you'll get a ballpark figure.

What do the test results mean?

If you're over age 21 with total cholesterol below 200, you're probably safe, most experts say.

Between 200 and 240, you have borderline high cholesterol. A large study found that, compared to men in the safe range, those in the borderline range have about twice the risk of death from heart disease. And there's no reason to believe that women with a similar lifestyle wouldn't have the same risk. Get rechecked at a hospital or clinical lab certified by, for example, the American College of Pathology or the Centers for Disease Control.

Above 240, you've officially got a dangerously high blood cholesterol level. In this range, men have about three times the risk of death from heart disease, according to the same study cited above. Have your total cholesterol, LDL, HDL, and triglycerides measured. This test costs more, around $15 to $30.

For best protection, LDL (low-density lipoprotein, the "bad" cholesterol) should be below 140 in men aged 40 to 59 and 118 in women of the same age group. The total cholesterol-to-HDL ratio should be less than 4.6 (which means 4.6 to 1) for men, less than 4.0 for women. Triglyceride levels should be less than 120 in men, lower in women.

Have any substances been debunked as cholesterol-busters?

Alcohol, once thought to raise HDL, is linked to obesity, high blood pressure, high triglycerides, and low HDLs. "We don't recommend alcohol to increase HDL," says Dr. Connor. "It doesn't work."

What's the best way to raise HDLs?

Dr. Cooper and other experts say aerobic exercise best raises HDL. Put diet to work, too. Once you've reduced your total fat intake, concentrate on substituting mostly monounsaturated fats (such as olive oil) for mostly polyunsaturated fats, which lower HDL, recommends Dr. Bonanome.

Is "hardening of the arteries" the result of plaque (cholesterol) buildup or a preexisting condition that primes arteries to collect cholesterol?

Scientists agree cholesterol causes hardening of the arteries, not vice versa. First, cholesterol accumulates in fatty yellow streaks on the walls of large arteries. This cholesterol builds up to form plaque, which narrows and hardens arteries. In time, a blood clot can lodge in the narrowed artery, stopping blood flow and causing a heart attack.

How good are the older cholesterol drugs?

Most people with high cholesterol don't need drugs. For them, diet is the preferred treatment. But for those with cholesterol over 300, cholestyramine (sold under the brand name Questran) and colestipol (Colestid) can work well. "They're generally safe, and ought to be used first before other drugs in most cases," says Dr. Connor.

In one study, cholestyramine reduced fatal heart disease by 24 percent. Colestipol is similarly effective. Combined with niacin, it reverses heart disease in some cases. But the drugs' sandy texture—and the constipation they sometimes cause—can make them hard to take.

Is the new drug lovastatin (Mevacor) as good as it sounds?

Lovastatin lowers cholesterol more than older drugs. Caution is essential, however. "The main problem is that one is embarking on a lifetime of therapy, and we don't know the long-term, possibly toxic, effects," says Dr. Connor.

In the short run, lovastatin can, in rare cases, cause inflamed muscles and liver problems. Eye exams are recommended to check for cataracts. Doctors agree that children and pregnant women generally shouldn't take it.

But lovastatin has doctors excited about the future. "It controls the liver, which manufactures 60 to 80 percent of the cholesterol in the blood," says Dr. Cooper. "Long term, that may be the answer; I'm not convinced this medication is it."

Eye Exercises for Better Vision

For Kay Connors, reading was a pain in the neck—literally. Ever since grade school, reading had given her eyestrain, headaches, and neck muscles tight as banjo strings.

"I felt incapable of reading, understanding, and retaining," she says. "I never read more than 20 minutes at a time." Over the years, Connors saw three ophthalmologists. Two said her vision was fine. The third prescribed reading glasses. But her neck pain persisted.

Then, at age 40, Connors went to an optometrist. He diagnosed convergence insufficiency: One of Connors's eyes wandered. Keeping her eyes aligned for reading took tremendous effort. The optometrist prescribed an eye-exercise treatment called vision therapy. Thanks to vision therapy, says Connors, a 45-year-old accountant and student, she now reads comfortably for hours at a time.

Connors's experience is not necessarily unique. Optometrists (O.D.'s trained to treat only vision) report vision therapy can resolve not only convergence insufficiency but also vision problems such as eye-shifting (fixation), focus-adjusting (accommodation), crossed eyes (strabismus), and lazy eyes (amblyopia). Nearsightedness (myopia), which affects 30 percent of us, may also be helped by this therapy, they claim. According to several optometrists interviewed, the therapy allows some people with small amounts of nearsightedness to do without glasses.They assert that even highly myopic people can reduce their prescriptions.

The Theory behind the Therapy

Vision therapy is based on the theory that, to a large extent, vision is learned. So a few vision therapists say that proper relearning can actually improve vision. Others say that the therapy simply helps eyes work more accurately or efficiently.

"Cross-eye," for example, is learned, claim vision therapists. An infant in a crib shoved against a wall, for instance, might learn to use one eye more than the other. A baby who sees only an unstimulating wall on one side will use that eye less.

"If they have experiences with only one eye, there's no way they'll learn to use their eyes together," says Donald Getz, O.D., 1987 chairman of the American Optometric Association's (AOA) vision training committee. The result: sometimes, a cross- or walleye.

And that's where vision therapy is supposed to help. After all, if poor vision is the result of poor training, then with proper retraining we can learn to see better, say optometrists who use vision therapy.

But vision therapy is not without controversy. No well-controlled studies support some claims made for it. And ophthalmologists (M.D.'s who specialize in treating eye diseases) say that many alleged improvements in eyesight after vision therapy come from patients wanting and expecting results—the common placebo effect.

Ophthalmologists question not only the claims but the theory behind the therapy. Anatomy and heredity, not learning, cause most myopia, they say. In myopia, the eyeball is too long or the cornea too curved, focusing light in front of the retina instead of on it—and no amount of relearning can change this. As for cross-eye, it's sometimes caused by premature birth, say ophthalmologists, but not by spending infancy in a crib up against a wall.

Still, there is some evidence that chronic close-focusing increases myopia, says Paul Vinger, M.D., assistant clinical professor of ophthalmology at Harvard University. And ophthalmologists admit research shows that vision therapy is effective in at least a few cases. It works in lazy eye, some types of cross-eye, some rare cases of myopia caused by "accommodative spasm" (eye muscles too tense to focus properly), and some convergence, fixation, and accommodative problems.

But what's vision therapy like?

Exercises for the Well-Trained Eye

One vision-therapy technique prescribed for myopia is the "body rock." To do it, patients use a wall calender. Taking off their glasses, patients stand far enough away so some numbers are clear. They rock forward on their feet until all the numbers are clear. Then they rock back until the numbers blur.

With practice, optometrists say, patients learn to relax their eye muscles enough to focus from the back position. How long this takes varies. Some people respond in 10 minutes, they say. Others take three weeks.

For patients with cross-eye, an optometrist might prescribe therapy with the "Marsden ball," a grapefruit-size ball that hangs from the ceiling on a string. The optometrist flashes a bright horizontal bar of light in the right eye and a vertical bar of light in the left. When both eyes aim properly at the ball, the patient sees afterimages of the bars overlapping in a cross. Eventually, patients get used to using their eyes together and do it unconsciously, optometrists say.

Lazy eye (dim sight in an eye) often accompanies cross-eye. It occurs when the brain suppresses vision in one eye as a way of compensating for the confusion of each eye seeing different things. Sometimes simply putting a patch over the dominant eye makes the other work harder. Another exercise requires tape, cardboard, a paper-towel tube, a 100-watt frosted light bulb, and a flashing-light socket (plug flasher). Under the supervision of an optometrist, patients tape cardboard across the end of the tube to form a cross. After plugging the light bulb into the flasher, patients cover the good eye, hold the bulb at the end of the tube, and look at the flashing light through the tube for about a minute. This creates an after-image of the cross on the fovea, the part of the eye that sees best and which the brain is suppressing. Then patients try to aim the afterimage at a target and hold it there. Aiming and holding the afterimage teaches patients where the fovea is and how to aim the eye more accurately.

Controversies in Vision Training

Among vision therapists' most controversial claims is that vision therapy betters athletic performance. Some professional teams subscribe to the idea, though. A football player hoping to make the Super Bowl-champion Washington Redskins has to make the grade with the team's vision therapists, Ronald Berger, O.D., and Harry Wachs, O.D. If visual skills don't meet Redskins' standards, the player has less chance of making the team.

Vision therapy isn't just for pros, optometrists say. "The weekend athlete who can't keep his eye on the ball can definitely improve," says Carl Gruning, O.D., a member of the AOA Council on Clinical Optometric Care. "Like most people, he likely has mild instability in eye coordination, focusing, or movement." A tennis player, for instance, can learn to see the ball when it comes off an opponent's racket, instead of when it crosses the net, he says.

To teach quicker reflexes, optometrists use a saccadic

(pronounced *sah-KAD-ik,* meaning eye movement) fixator, a board studded with lights. Picture a Chinese-checkers board with dozens of lights where the holes would be. Across the room from the device, patients hit a button each time a light flashes. With practice, hands and eyes respond more quickly to the flashing lights, reducing reaction time. Quicker reactions with the saccadic fixator lead to quicker reactions on the court, say optometrists.

Still more controversial are some optometrists' claims of reforming juvenile delinquents. Delinquency, they say, often results from learning problems caused by poor vision. Correct the underlying vision problems and delinquents usually go straight, say optometrists.

As with other claims for vision therapy, controlled studies of its effects on juvenile delinquents are lacking. The connection between vision therapy and improved reading is equally tenuous, ophthalmologists say. In 1984, the American Academy of Ophthalmology issued a statement saying, "No known scientific evidence supports claims for improving academic abilities . . . or modification of delinquent or criminal behavior with treatment based on vision training . . . . "

So how do ophthalmologists explain stories about improvements in the behavior of delinquents treated with vision therapy? They say delinquents may act better simply because they're getting attention.

Ophthalmologists are equally dubious of vision therapy's impact on athletic performance. "If there were an Olympics for saccadic fixators, training athletes on them would be great," says Dr. Vinger. "But can getting fast on a saccadic fixator make you hit a tennis ball better? It's unproven."

Ophthalmologists don't rule out the possibility that vision therapy might reform delinquents, improve athletes, and do everything else optometrists claim. But the burden of proof is on the optometrists. And so far, ophthalmologists say, the proof isn't in.

Is Vision Therapy for You?

Optometrists themselves say vision therapy can't treat every eye problem. It doesn't cure presbyopia, the near-point fuzziness that strikes virtually everyone over age 40. And, unless you have other symptoms—eyestrain, watery eyes, headaches, and poor depth perception or peripheral vision— don't get vision therapy for farsightedness. It isn't a well-established treatment, even in the eyes of optometrists.

Nor can vision therapy treat eye diseases like glaucoma and cataracts. If you have disease symptoms—double vision, sudden loss of vision in one eye, bulging eyeball, drooping eyelid, one pupil bigger than the other, pain, redness, discharge, flashes of light, sudden appearance of "floaters"—see an ophthalmologist. You need an M.D.'s attention.

But if you share Kay Connors' convergence problem or have any of the conditions described earlier for which vision training offers some promise, you may want to consider this unconventional approach. If you do, keep the following in mind.

Cost • Approach the cost of vision therapy with open eyes. Most health insurance plans cover it, but if yours doesn't, therapy can be expensive. Eight months of once-a-week therapy may run from $1,200 to $2,000.

Time and Commitment • Vision training requires time and patience. You can't expect results unless you practice. Can you stick with an exercise program? If so, then you're likely to give vision therapy a good shot. If not, don't even consider it.

Qualified Instruction • Consult an optometrist who regularly practices vision therapy. Most don't. You can find the certified practitioner nearest you by writing or calling the College of Optometrists in Vision Development at P.O. Box 285, Chula Vista, CA 92012-0285 (619) 425-6191.

The Healing
Power
of Walking

Giving Your Ticker
a Tune-Up

Walking is wonderful: It's the exercise that doesn't feel like exercise. And while most of us know that walking is good for us, we may not know just how good. Sure, walking is an "aerobic" exercise; it strengthens the heart. But did you know that it can add several years to your life in terms of heart health? And while it's obvious that walking can burn calories, you may not know it can sculpt your body to svelte proportions!

Turn Back the Clock

Walking can't reverse time (not even if you walk backward), but it can make your heart beat as if you were years younger. The best evidence of the heart-protecting power of exercise like walking comes from a pair of studies done by Lars G. Ekelund, M.D., Ph.D., an associate professor of medicine at the University of North Carolina at Chapel Hill. In one study, Dr. Ekelund and his colleagues put 3,106 healthy men between the ages of 30 and 69 through a treadmill test. Each man was assigned a "fitness rating" based on his heart rate during exercise and the length of time he was able to stay on the treadmill. Over the next $8\frac{1}{2}$ years, 45 of those men died from cardiovascular disease. After adjusting for other risk factors—age, smoking, HDL cholesterol, and blood pressure—the researchers confirmed that a low level of fitness is itself a major independent risk factor for heart attack and stroke (*New England Journal of Medicine*).

Men aren't the only ones who raise their risks of heart disease each time they lower their fanny into a recliner. Dr. Ekelund's second fitness study investigated women's risks.

This second study was similar to the first: 2,802 women (ages 30 to 69) were followed for $10\frac{1}{2}$ years; 40 died of heart disease. Once again, a lower level of treadmill-tested fitness was associated with greatly increased risk of death independent of other risk factors, such as diabetes, high blood pressure, and smoking (*Circulation*).

This means that "couch potatoes" face the same risk of heart disease as pack-a-day smokers or people with 300-plus cholesterol levels. Further, extrapolating from his data, Dr. Ekelund explains that not exercising is like tacking many years of wear and tear on the heart! In effect, it ages you. But a simple program of aerobic-type exercise—such as walking for about 30 minutes three times a week—can reclaim those "lost" years. It's an awfully easy way to lengthen your life.

Walk Away from Risk Boosters

Beyond boosting cardiovascular fitness, walking seems to protect the heart in other ways. For starters, regular exercise like walking may raise HDLs (high-density lipoproteins), the "good" kind of cholesterol. Fitness walking may also lower LDLs (low-density lipoproteins), the artery-clogging cholesterol, and triglycerides. You won't see these important benefits with an ordinary finger-stick test that measures total cholesterol.

But doctors now say that the higher your HDL level—and the lower your cholesterol-to-HDL ratio (that is, the total cholesterol number divided by HDL)—the better your chances of avoiding heart disease.

Brisk walking also helps lower blood pressure. In recent studies linking exercise with blood pressure, James Hagberg, Ph.D., a researcher at the National Institute on Aging, found that exercisers had an average 20-point drop in their systolic blood pressure and a 10-point drop in their diastolic after completing an exercise program. That could make a big difference to someone with borderline high blood pressure!

Body Sculpting: Slim Down and Trim Up

Meanwhile, for those of us who want to look as good on the outside as we feel on the inside, walking offers additional benefits. First, as we've said many times before, walking is your best low-impact exercise for weight loss. "Mile for mile, jogging burns only about 20 percent more calories than brisk walking," says James M. Rippe, M.D., associate professor of medicine at the University of Massachusetts Medical Center in Worcester. Plus, walking off your calories carries less chance of joint injury than jogging.

Best of all, through walking you'll lose weight in all the right places—not just on the legs but also on the abdomen, hips, upper arms—wherever you've got too much fat. Surprised? Don't be. Walking is an aerobic activity, which means it burns off body fat. And usually the areas of highest fat concentration melt away first. In men, that usually means the gut; in women, the hips and thighs. The good news is that you can burn off much of that fat!

"It won't all go away overnight. And some people won't take off as much as they'd like to in certain areas," explains Charles Eichenberg, Ph.D., director of the New Start Health Center in St. Petersburg, Florida. "But for most of us, regular walking will make visible changes."

The sculpting effect isn't all due to fat loss. Walking tones up muscles, too—and again the legs aren't the only beneficiaries. "Walking is a carefully designed balancing act. The muscles of the abdomen and lower back can get a moderate workout just keeping your trunk in line with your legs during a brisk walk. That's how you keep moving forward without falling flat on your face," says Randall L. Braddom, M.D., director of physical medicine and rehabilitation at Providence Hospital in Cincinnati.

Your arms and upper torso get a mild to moderate workout when you walk, because you naturally swing your arms. You can increase that workout by deliberately pumping your arms. That also helps you pick up the pace. And if you really want to strengthen your upper body as you walk, you can use hand-held weights. (Two pounds per hand is sufficient.) Properly used, the weights won't cause injury, and they can increase the aerobic value of your workout while toning your arms.

Slow and Steady

Walking can work wonders for your health and body image, but you've got to stick with it. Regular workouts are the key. And you have to keep your expectations in pace with your workouts. "If it took you 40 years to get the body shape you have today, you can't expect to reverse the process in 40 days," says James Stray-Gundersen, M.D., assistant professor of surgery and physiology at the University of Texas Southwestern Medical Center. "Nature does things best gradually."

So stick with it, and feel yourself growing stronger.

Get in Step with Someone You Love

You already know this: If you're having trouble sticking with your walking program, finding a partner may help you stay motivated. And science confirms it. Fifty-one men enrolled in a hospital-based exercise program at St. Francis Medical Center in Peoria, Illinois, were twice as likely to stick with their walking programs for a year if their wives also exercised.

But you may not be fully aware of this: Walking, in often subtle ways, can help build relationships. If, for example, you're having trouble finding quiet time to communicate with a special person in your life, scheduling walking time together could solve that problem—and give you both the benefits of exercise to boot.

Cynthia Strowbridge, a New York City psychotherapist, encourages clients to walk together, especially if they've been experiencing tension in the relationship.

"The tension can be dispersed through the exercise, rather than channeled into an outburst of emotion," says Strowbridge. "And walking together can often ease communication in another way. It's natural to have silent pauses while you walk. Those same pauses in a more sedentary setting can be awkward and anxiety-producing."

Walking toward Communication

We tend to think of communicating strictly in terms of talking. But have you ever walked in silence with someone close to you and felt a strong feeling of connection?

"We forget how intimate it is to be wholeheartedly with another person in silence. Being in step together, outdoors, can be amazingly healing to body and spirit."

It may be easier to experience this silent connectedness while walking because, in part, going for a walk together gets you away from distractions like TV, telephones, and household demands.

Jerilyn Ross, associate director of the Roundhouse Square Psychiatric Center and president of the Phobia Society of America, feels even more strongly about walking to enhance relationships since she started her nightly jaunts with her brother.

"We were having trouble getting together to just talk. We're both night owls, so after his family is in bed and my work is done, he walks to my house (about $1\frac{1}{2}$ miles), we walk back to his house, and he drives me home. We talk and get exercise, too.

"Couples, family members, and close friends have so little time to be together without disruptions," says Ross. "Setting aside time to be together without distraction enhances your sense of commitment to each other."

Easing the Aches and Pains of Arthritis

Most of us are probably familiar with the old Henny Youngman joke about the patient who tells the doctor, "Hey, Doc, it hurts when I do this," and the doctor responds, "Then don't do that!" But for people with arthritis, it's no joke. They respond to achy joints just that way, not realizing that lack of movement can compound the problem.

Once properly diagnosed and treated (with appropriate medication, if needed, and physical therapy), most people with arthritis can benefit from a regular exercise program, says rheumatologist Sam Schatten, M.D., of Atlanta, Georgia. Recent research suggests that walking may be the best exercise for them.

Walking helps to strengthen the muscles around the joints. This in turn may prevent joint injury and disfigurement and seems to relieve some of the pain that may occur when bones rub against bones.

The natural tranquilizing effect of walking also helps to ease arthritis pain. And its mood-elevating effect offers an added benefit.

"Walking can greatly improve a person's attitude and fight the vicious circle of depression and pain," says Dr. Schatten.

Gale Snyder knows this all too well. A schoolteacher and mother of two who's had rheumatoid arthritis for four years, she finds that walking eases her pain and depression like nothing else. "I feel terrible when I'm sitting and feeling stiff. That hurts more than moving," Snyder says. "Plus, walking is a great stress reliever for me. I can cope with my fears so much better after a good walk. And I found that when I listen to music on a walk, I get a rush of good feeling—of feeling strong and powerful." In fact, she shared her enthusiasm for walking to music by creating the first aerobic walking tape, called "Walktime."

Kate Lorig, Doctor of Public Health, of the Stanford University Arthritis Center, endorses walking for arthritis management. "In addition to increasing muscle and joint strength and reducing depression, walking helps bone maintain calcium," she says.

At the Stanford Center, Dr. Lorig encourages patients to use their common sense to develop a personalized walking regimen. "I tell people to start slowly, walking as far as they can without feeling more pain than before they started. If that means walking across the room, fine. One block or two blocks? That's a good start," she says.

It's very important for arthritics to listen to their body. "Pain is a valuable indicator of misuse," Dr. Lorig adds. "Although arthritics may experience some pain with any movement, if the pain worsens when they begin to walk, they may be damaging their joints. Strengthening or stretching exercises—or perhaps some medication—may be needed. It's very important to work with your physician.

"Some people fear that their pain might flare up on a long walk, leaving them stranded. I remind them that they can walk 5 miles and never be more than a half block from home if they just walk up and down the street," Dr. Lorig says.

Once a person has established the distance he or she can comfortably walk, Dr. Lorig suggests getting into a routine. Walk three to four times a week, increasing your distance by no more than 10 percent every two weeks, she says.

Keep in mind, too, that your walking program has to remain flexible. If pain or inflammation flares up, trim your schedule, even put your fitness program on hold for a few days. "This isn't a setback," says Dr. Lorig. "Consider it an integral part of your overall plan for pain management."

Walking in Water

For some arthritics, even the gentlest exercise can cause discomfort. If that sounds like your situation, consider this soothing alternative: aquatic exercise. It's not water ballet, but it is an excellent way to improve and maintain joint flexibility and increase muscle strength. The water displaces body weight, putting less stress on the joints. There is also a kind of external massagelike effect, and the water offers enough resistance to strengthen the muscles. And because exercising in the water is less painful, people are more likely to do it on a regular basis.

The Arthritis Foundation and the YMCA cosponsor water exercise programs around the country. Classes led by a qualified instructor meet at least once a week. People find the social atmosphere of a water workout to be supportive and encouraging.

At the YMCA in Bethlehem, Pennsylvania, for example, a group of about 30 men and women meet three days a week for range-of-motion exercises and walking in the pool. For some, this is their only form of exercise. For others, this is part of a fitness program that also includes regular walks on land. Says Doris Transue of Hellertown, Pennsylvania, "The social atmosphere of the classes really helps. And because of the classes, I don't have to work out on a resistance machine anymore."

For more information on an aquatics program near you, contact your local Arthritis Foundation, YMCA or YWCA.

Slow and Steady Wins the Race

Scientists are impressed, and walkers are delighted: Unwanted pounds are coming off and staying off for good, to the steady beat of walking feet. But why? What makes walking so tough on unwanted pudge?

Speed Is Not of the Essence • As obesity experts point out, one of the most common pitfalls of starting an exercise program is trying to do too much too soon. "Many people have an all-or-nothing attitude about exercise," points out bariatric physician Scott Rigden, M.D. But walking offers a wide range of acceptable paces—from a slow stroll for starters to a brisk arm-pumping stride later on.

Walking burns calories at any speed. Of course, brisker walking burns more. But if you can't (or don't want to) go faster, you can walk longer to make up the difference. For example, if you weigh 150 pounds and cover 1 mile in 15 minutes (that's 4 mph), you burn about 110 calories. But walk at a slower (3 mph) pace and you get the same calorie burn in just 1$\frac{1}{10}$ mile. "This is truly a race that the tortoise wins, not the hare," says cardiologist and walking expert James Rippe, M.D.

Walking Powers Up Your Cells • Increased calorie burning that happens during your walk continues for a while after your walk is over. But you may not realize that this short "afterburn" can, in a sense, turn into a "continual burn."

That's because regular walking signals the muscle cells to increase the size and number of mitochondria—the structures that help burn up calories, as engines burn gasoline. So the more you walk, the more engines you build to burn increasing amounts of calories. Your "fuel guzzling" is faster and may go on for hours and hours. "We're talking about a Ferrari compared with a Volkswagen," says Peter D. Wood, Ph.D., a professor of medicine and fitness expert.

Walking Alters the Fuel Mix • Your body uses up more fat for energy once you become a walker. Why? Two reasons. First, walking increases the concentration of oxidative enzymes in your cells. These enzymes are needed for fat metabolism. "Exercising improves the body's ability to use body fat for fuel," says Herman M. Frankel, M.D.

Second, walkers employ the so-called slow-twitch, rather than fast-twitch, muscles. A bird that flies the Atlantic Ocean has slow-twitch muscles in its wings. Your legs have them, too. And guess what—the mitochondria in slow-twitch muscle fibers prefer fat. "Muscles designed to do long, continuous movements tend to be the fat-burning type of muscle," says Dr. Wood.

Walking Makes You Thinner All Over • You'd expect walking to trim and tone your legs. And it does. But the flab-trimming may not stop there. A study at the University of California reported "a striking loss of fat over the arm" in both walkers and cyclists after six months of regular exercise (*American Journal of Sports Medicine*). Walking can take off fat anywhere—from jelly belly to thunder thighs, claims the study's chief investigator, Grant Gwinup, M.D.

Walkers Hold On to Lean Body Mass • When you diet without exercising, up to 30 percent of every pound you lose may be muscle. And not just any old muscle. A recent study showed that even valuable heart muscle was lost when dieters did not exercise.

Beat feet, however, and you lose lard and only lard. It's true—the pounds you drop can be pure pudge, which leaves you with more muscle per square inch than when you started.

Muscle looks better. It takes up less room, so your clothes feel looser. And muscle burns more calories than fat does, even when you're asleep.

Walking More Lets You Eat More • You've heard it a million times: Exercise regularly and you'll slim down. Very true. But did you know that you'll be able to eat up? Once they've reached goal weight, walkers eat more than nonwalkers—yet stay trimmer. Think about that next time you're tempted to skip your walk.

Diet or not, you'll walk off excess pounds. Maintain a constant food intake and you'll lose weight slowly. (Walk 45 minutes a day, four times a week, and you could drop almost 18 pounds in a year.) Snip out a few hundred calories per day and the pounds will leave faster. Either way, you'll be much less hungry—and better nourished—than someone who cuts calories drastically.

Walking Sidesteps the "I've Gotta Eat" Blues • Many people put on extra pounds by using food to deal with stress and tension. A bowl of ice cream subs as a tranquilizer. But while high-fat goodies travel straight to your hips and set up house there, a walk takes you way beyond the tension of the moment.

In a study at the University of Massachusetts Center for Health and Fitness, researchers found that walking reduces anxiety, no matter how casual or intense the workout. And this calming effect lasts for at least 2 hours after exercise.

Walking Goes Easy on the Joints • Walking is the sport that's custom-made for folks with lots of excess poundage. That's because it's ever so gentle, even on the back, hips, knees and ankles—prime trouble spots for overweight people.

And walking in shallow water is even gentler. "This really saves the lower joints and helps osteoarthritis," says Dr. Rigden. Water has a buoyant effect, yet offers resistance that helps tone muscles and burn fat.

So walk, stroll or stride—you're on your way to a stronger, leaner shape!

WALKING FOR WEIGHT LOSS— AND A WHOLE LOT MORE

Here are two pounds-off stories with healthy endings. Many people walk to lose weight. But for some, weight loss isn't the ultimate goal; it's the means to achieve something more—good health. Two cases in point: Robin Simon and Bob Grohne. Overweight and suffering from disabling illnesses, they each discovered the remarkable benefits of walking. Here they tell how they took weight loss—and health recovery—in stride.

Robin Simon, Whitefish, Montana

"It didn't happen overnight. Years of stress-induced eating, after-work snacking, second helpings, and no exercise left me 55 pounds overweight.

"I wouldn't admit I was fat. I never looked in a full-length mirror. I liked to think of myself as being big-boned and pretended to disguise the fat behind oversized clothing I sewed for myself (no size labels inside!).

"After marriage, babies and baking became my favorite hobbies and I assured myself that I could lose weight if I really wanted to.

"The excruciating pain of a ruptured disk convinced me that perhaps now was the time. I was confined to bed for several months and faced back surgery. For the first

(continued)

time in my life I took a serious look at myself and made up my mind to lose weight.

"I went on a diet and managed to lose 30 pounds before the operation. But I had another 20 to go after the surgery. My doctor suggested daily walking in order to recover fully. I literally had to learn to walk all over again.

"At first I could manage only $\frac{1}{2}$ mile a day, but I soon worked up to 2 miles. The pounds melted off and in no time at all I reached my goal.

"With less weight to carry around, I felt more energetic and self-confident. I began setting higher walking goals for myself. I now try to walk 25 miles a week. Sometimes I challenge myself to see how far or how fast I can go. Walking supplies me with a feeling of control over my body. I can tune in and experience my heart beating faster and my lungs working harder as I climb a hill or increase my speed. It's a great feeling.

"Walking helped me to discover a wealth of personal power to draw from. It took a major obstacle to get me to accept the challenge, but meeting the challenge has meant countless benefits. I'm living proof that walking can help a person succeed in losing weight."

Bob Grohne, Decatur, Illinois

"At 6 feet in height and 330 pounds, I qualified as 'gorilla' on most life-insurance medical charts. Happiness was a warm bowl of potato chips and a good football game on the tube.

"Thirty years in heavy construction taught me how to drink three pots of coffee per day and then calm down on an equal number of packs of cigarettes. Other than setting the office wastebasket on fire now and then, no great damage seemed to have been done.

"Then a funny thing happened.

"After a nasty conference with the local business agent for the union, I went back to the office to calm down with another cup of coffee and the ever-present cigarette. The funny thing was not being able to find the end of the cigarette to light. My hand seemed to be missing, too. Blank!

"I woke up in the intensive-care unit with hoses going in and out, machines going 'huckey-puckey' and a group dressed in white gathered around my bed looking grim.

(continued)

WALKING FOR WEIGHT LOSS—*Continued*

"I had had a simultaneous stroke and heart attack, which brought on locked kidneys, a blood pressure reading of 280 over 220, and a loss of eyesight. I had some peripheral vision, but the rest was as though someone had popped a flashbulb at close range.

"On my sixth day of hospitalization, a beam of hope came skipping into the room. An old buddy of mine, flashing his Baptist minister's pass to the head nurse, parked his sweat suit next to my bed.

" 'First,' he said, 'get yourself out of here. Then try walking to get some of this blubber off you. We'll do it together.'

"Three years later, 80 pounds of that blubber has evaporated. My blood pressure has fallen back to a controllable range, my eyesight is 20-20, there's no sign of heart problems, and my kidneys are doing their thing.

"In the beginning, I could barely walk one block before sitting down and puffing like a wounded water buffalo. With my friend's prodding, I worked up to 1 mile, then 2. By the end of the summer, we did a 14-mile stint together, although we wanted to die afterward!

"The conquistadors may not have found the fountain of youth, but had they kept walking, I think the net effect would have been the same. I have a body that renewed itself at age 55.

"Slimmer and more toned than ever before, I plan to continue walking to keep my body in shape."

The Practical Psychology of Positive Living

What It Means to Follow Your Dreams

By Dennis T. Jaffe, Ph.D., and Cynthia D. Scott, Ph.D.

What makes you want to come to work each day? There's a story about three stonecutters in a large courtyard, each cutting stones with a chisel. A stranger wandered up to them and asked what they were doing. The first one replied curtly, "Can't you see I'm cutting stones?" The stranger moved away quickly and approached the second stonecutter. He again asked, "What are you doing?" The second man replied warmly, "I'm working so that my family can live and grow." The stranger then queried the third cutter, who replied with a swelling sense of pride, "I'm building a cathedral. Each stone I cut goes into a house of worship that will last far beyond my life."

Each of these workers performed the same task. But how different the work felt to each of them! The first worker felt tired, exhausted, and bored by his work because he was unable to see the larger picture. The second felt satisfaction, even enthusiasm, because he could see what his work would bring to him. The third cutter saw his work connected to a larger whole, full of spiritual meaning and significance. His mundane toil was accompanied by a vision of what his stones would become and how they would enrich other people's lives. This cutter was connected to his inner mission and had a vision of why he was working.

Which of these three workers are you most like? What is the personal meaning of your own work? What do you first think of when you think of your mission and your vision of life? Do you imagine that what you really want to achieve is beyond your reach? May never happen? Is not realistic or practical?

People who follow a dream or have a deep sense of purpose about their work are rewarded with an almost inexhaustible supply of energy. They use this energy to reach their goals. Burned-out people have lost their sense of purpose; their work no longer matters to them. Many of them have, in effect, retired on the job.

Several things cause this state of affairs. One is a shift in what your job means to you. When you enter a new profession, one of the major motivators is the desire to demonstrate excellence. In the first years of work, you develop your skills and begin to experience their rewards. In addition to the external reward of money and status, you have the inner reward of feeling good about doing well. Somewhere along the way, your motivation to be competent can waver. At this point, people report that their work is getting routine, that it does not have the kick anymore.

The challenge now is to shift from the motivation of learning more new things to something else. Many people at midcareer switch from motivation by competence to motivation according to inner meaning—from the "how" to the "why." People seek meaningful relationships, a sense of purpose, a feeling of community with coworkers. Workers want to be valued for what they are, not just what they can do. In our study of 450 physicians in transition, the major finding was that physicians were changing their work styles so they could feel more connected to the ancient tradition of the healer and were rejecting the emphasis on purely technological medicine.

Feeling part of something larger than themselves, people give their best. The more of themselves they invest, the more exciting, energizing, and fulfilling work becomes. However, no one can just command investment in work. There has to be an inner reason for this commitment. That inner meaning comes from the individual's and the company's mission, vision, or purpose.

First You Dream

Think about your mission. What do you think about first? You might think of something deeply meaningful to you, such as, "I want to improve the quality of life," or "I want to help young children learn to read," or "I want to make cities better places to live." People with a mission experience a real drive for what they do, especially when they can feel that their actions now contribute to the mission. Contrast the energy and commitment of people who work on political campaigns, putting in 16-hour days ringing doorbells because they believe their candidate can make a real difference, with employees who are asked to do similar tasks as part of a market survey for a product they think is useless.

Think of your mission not as a solid, unchangeable road but as a garden in which your activities develop. All your tasks may seem very different, but when brought together in the garden they all relate to each other. In a garden, each plant is distinct, and no one plant makes a garden, but together all the plants form an interrelated whole. In the same way, no one activity is enough to fulfill your mission. Defining your own inner mission—envisioning your garden—is the first step to maintaining and growing your energy.

On a piece of paper, make a list of the things you want in your life. You might divide the paper into two sides, one side for work and one for personal/family life. Make the list as long as you can. Include specific things like "I want to manage a new-product campaign," as well as more general ones like "I want to contribute to world peace."

Think of the items on this list as the individual plants in your garden. You can discover your mission (your overall visions and your values) by seeing what groups from your list have in common—in other words, what patterns exist in your garden. For example, you might find that several of your wants relate to helping people learn and grow, so that is a major value for you.

The blossoms and fruits of the plants are the specific activities you do each day to move toward these goals. Take one of your wants, perhaps something like, "being recognized as an important contributor to my profession." Now think about some immediate and some longer-term things you could do to move toward this. Eventually, you can create a blossom for each of your wants, with specific actions.

Defining your mission acts as an emotional touchstone that unleashes a powerful feeling. You might recognize a hidden dream that has been buried for a long time because someone once said it was silly.

One way to explore your hidden dreams is to remember the roles you have thought about and your role models for them. If you want to be a newscaster, singer, or executive, for example, what particular person is most like the person you would like to be? What aspect of this person's life is your goal? Would it be the glamour and publicity, the acclaim for performances, the ability to make decisions that touch many people's lives, or the opportunity to be seen as an authority? There may be very different reasons for each dream role, leading to very different touchstones.

Finding What You Stand For

Values form the building blocks of your mission. So one way to craft a mission for yourself is to explore your values—the things that you personally stand for.

Values form the core of your understanding about the world, the basis for your deepest feelings. They act as motivators for your beliefs and actions. You can also think of them as the main themes upon which you weave the experiences of your life. Values feed your passion for the activities that you undertake over the long run. They do not usually change drastically throughout your life but act as an anchor, allowing you to return to your original purpose when off base.

Your core values tell what you stand for. Many of us, unfortunately, have grown up with the sense that values are like rules—straitjackets that limit our behavior. Yet when we look at people who deeply believe in something, we see the opposite. We see people who can draw on vast reserves of energy that seem to flow from their beliefs.

Values are an energy source. A person who believes in something, who acts on what seems really important, always finds the energy to accomplish the task. People disconnected from this energy source find themselves struggling against burnout.

Psychologist Douglas LaBier, in *Modern Madness: The Emotional Fallout of Success,* writes about the pain of executives who pursue success and end up betraying their inner values. These young men pursue the traditional outer-directed path to wealth, status, and success, only to find an inner emptiness and worthlessness. They reach a crisis of meaning. Their resolution of this upheaval is a new orientation to work in concert with inner values, and they pursue a clearer vision of what is really important to them. Often, this vision was clearer to them when they were younger, but the pressures of getting ahead at work pushed it to the back burner as they told themselves it was unrealistic or impractical. Now they find that reconnecting to their mission is critical to their well-being.

One step in finding your own mission through values is to use an imagery technique. To begin, take some time to get relaxed. Take a deep breath, clearing your mind of all the thoughts and everyday concerns you are carrying. Now ask yourself the questions, "What do I stand for? What are my deepest personal values?" Hold that thought and let your unconscious answer. You will probably get a number of responses.

Another way to ask the question is to think about what you would most want to teach your children. What is the most important lesson you have for them? Would it be truth, beauty, freedom, harmony? Allow yourself to formulate these values in any way that makes sense to you.

Now recall a time when you took a stand about your values. Allow yourself to re-create that situation. See yourself acting in accordance with your values. What does it feel like to act in this way? If you have more than one value, imagine them lining up. Take a moment to consider each one in sequence. Allow your mind to wander over all of them, and select one value that seems to be at the center of all your values.

Now let your imagination create a symbol that represents your value. It could be an object, a sound, a color, a smell, a texture, a person, or an animal. Be willing to be surprised by what your imagination produces. Just accept whatever comes to you. Do not be judgmental. This symbol will act as an anchor, bringing you back to this core value whenever you need it. Drawing a picture of your symbol will give you something to grab when you may have lost touch with your core value.

You may wonder: Why a picture? Images have a special quality: They give a shape and form to your value and can be used as an anchor when you want to return to them. They do more than just state a value; they add an emotional identification to an abstract concept. Symbols and pictures move you.

One woman whose basic value was in growing and being open to new experiences came up with the image of an acorn in her first imagery exercise. At first this seemed tiny and insignificant in relation to her large dreams for her life. What changed her understanding was looking more deeply into the image and seeing that the acorn has all the energy to blossom into a huge tree. She used the emotional feeling of the tiny acorn giving birth to the huge flowing tree to remind herself of the energy she had inside to accomplish her dreams. She found a tree branch and mounted it on her desk to remind herself that the big tree started as a dream of the acorn. This branch reminded her to connect her regular work activities with her own personal growth.

Hooking Your Mission onto Reality

Taking your sense of personal mission and combining it with your work is the big challenge. The initial step is to make your mission portable. Distill your mission into a few words. These words will act like an emotional touchstone, enabling you to remember your larger purpose in an instant.

Take a few moments right now to put your mission into a

short phrase. Ask yourself, "What is it about my mission that makes me most excited? Is it the creative fulfillment, the fame, the money, the chance to help people, the closeness to nature?" Find the kernel of meaning at the center of what you want to do. Some examples are "News that serves" for someone in publicity; "Creating harmony through training" for someone in a management-development company; "The best damn truck in America" for a worker in a truck-manufacturing company. A touchstone needs to be brief, and often exciting, because it takes people right back to their core mission. What have you come up with? These phrases become handles, which you can use to carry your mission into your everyday work. Take a moment right now to write down your phrase.

Now bring your mission down to earth. If you work in a company and your job seems fixed, try to reconceptualize it from the perspective of your ideal vision. What could your job be if you and the company would let it? Practicality follows visioning; too often we get practical before we let ourselves dream and create freely.

Musician/educator Robert Fritz observes that there is always a distance between an ideal and reality. Most people resolve the tension by letting go of the dream and thereby not dealing with the discomfort. He suggests, however, that inspired performers are those who are able to live with the tension and begin to move the reality toward the vision. You can do this by generating ways to make your visions real. If you try to accomplish something every day that moves you toward your vision, and you take time each day to congratulate yourself and feel good about this accomplishment, you will find yourself energized by your work toward your vision.

A person can be motivated by his or her current reality, the status quo, or by a vision of what can be. People connecting only to current reality are committed to a steady state. They are reactive; they settle for or accept the way things are. In contrast, the more you are motivated by a vision, the more you are stretching, risking, striving, and reaching. You are growing toward your vision, and you need to be creative because you are continually trying to make reality more like your vision.

Nip Tension in the Bud

By Mark Golin

Relax. Easier said than done, right? Even when you think you're relaxed, there may still be this insidious stream of tension coiling through your body. It's with you all the time. As a matter of fact, it's so subtle and constant, you may not even know it's there. So how do you get rid of something you can't find?

May I suggest a relaxation routine that makes you tense?

Believe it or not, "progressive relaxation" gets people to experience tension so they can recognize it, then defuse it when it crops up in real life.

Stress Times Two

According to experts, there are two types of stress. The first is immediate stress. It's that tense, edgy feeling you get while driving on an icy, dangerous road, for example. The body responds immediately and unmistakably—with faster breathing, tensed muscles, quickened heartbeat and more— then shifts back to normal as soon as the crisis has passed.

The second type—and the most insidious—is long-term stress. It's that deep uneasiness you feel when you've got some unresolved problem nagging at your mind. Even when you try to push the problem aside so you can get on with other matters, your brain is always aware of the conflict. Just as it hypes up your body to deal with an icy road, your brain rallies the body to deal with the underlying worry. The end result is a subtle, 24-hour-a-day state of tension. It's so gradual and so constant, you may not know it's there.

And, unfortunately, it's what you don't know that can hurt you. Experts say that the body's stress response is due, in part, to the release of hormones. For example, when the brain recognizes a crisis, it orders the release of the hormone adrenaline—a little biological trick originally designed to give us the ability to fight with more strength or run away like there's no tomorrow.

Fortunately, the short-term surge of hormones in reaction to stress is essentially harmless. But what is perfectly acceptable for the body in the short term becomes a chemical imbalance in the long run. Eventually, the weakest parts of the body may break down under this hormonal barrage. End result? The development of chronic stress-related disease.

Obviously, the best way to alleviate long-term stress is to resolve the underlying worry or mental conflict causing it. But let's face it, such inner problems are often tough to identify and deal with. Unraveling them may take time and effort, sometimes even psychological counseling. However, experts point out that the next best thing to eliminating the source of stress is reducing the tension that always follows it. That's what this routine is designed to do.

The Power of PR

Progressive relaxation (PR) can be a powerful weapon against hidden tension. For years, stress experts have recommended it as a way to train yourself to detect physical tension and to relax enough to squelch it.

When you master PR, you'll find yourself suddenly sensitive to previously unnoticed muscular tension—that slight shoulder tightness or that uneasiness in the back muscles. And by immediately doing the tension-relaxation exercises of PR, you'll be able to nip that tension in the bud.

Are you willing to give it a try? Good. Let's get started.

First, loosen your clothing, lower the lights, and take the phone off the hook (unexpected interruption is the patron saint of tension). Then lie down on a firm surface; I used the living-room floor.

Now take a breath. Not like the two or three thousand you take every day. Pull in a long, cool draft of air and let it out slowly and reluctantly. Do about five of these little refreshers, and don't be in a hurry to move on. For this technique to be worthwhile, a calm mind and concentration are important ingredients.

Now tense your muscles (and maintain the tension) in the following sequence, until your whole body is taut and strained: Clench your teeth. Squeeze your eyes shut. Make tight fists, and bring them up to your shoulders, contracting your arm muscles hard. Pull your stomach in toward your spine and straighten your legs. Dig your heels into the floor and clench your toes.

For at least 30 seconds hold this whole-body state of tension and mark it well. Really pay attention to how the strain and tightness feels in each muscle group. Let the tension build . . . and build . . . then release. Let your body go limp. Take a deep breath and appreciate the relaxation.

Now you know a little more about the difference between muscular tension and the rewarding sensation of relaxation. Just as a cool drink seems cooler after a hot one, so too will you better understand tension and relaxation by contrasting the two feelings.

Try this total-body tension routine a few times, giving yourself a good 2 minutes of deep breathing between attempts.

The next step is to try this tension/relaxation sequence on individual muscle groups, keeping all other muscles relaxed. Start with your hands. Hold them away from your body, then make fists. Clench them tight and hold for a count of five, noting the feeling of tension in the muscles. Then relax. Open your hands and wiggle your fingers, relishing the feeling of tension relief, of pure relaxation. Do this three times, slowly, allowing yourself time to concentrate on the contrasting sensations.

Then do your arms, one at a time. Just as you did in the full-body tense, make a fist and bring it up to your shoulder while flexing your arm muscles. Hold this position briefly, noting the tension. Then unclench the fist and let your arm fall back to a relaxed position, savoring the feeling of release. Do this three times with each arm, taking three to five deep, slow breaths after each tension-relaxation sequence.

Now you can try the same sequence on all the remaining major muscle groups, from head to toe. In each of the exercises listed below, remember to concentrate on the contrasting sensations you're feeling, and follow the same pattern of three repetitions that you used for the arms, taking slow breaths between reps. Only the part of the body you're working should feel tension.

- Forehead: Scrunch up your forehead. Feel those worry lines getting accentuated.
- Mouth: Open your mouth as wide as you can three times, then clench your jaw tightly by biting down hard.
- Shoulders: Shrug your shoulders, trying to touch your ears with them.
- Chest: Take a deep breath, completely filling your lungs. Pay particular attention to the tension in your ribs.
- Stomach: Push your stomach out as far as it will go, until you feel like a balloon ready to burst. Now take a moment and mentally feel out the body parts you've worked on. Any tension creeping back into them? If so, try a few more repetitions on them before moving on.
- Back: Lie down on your back and arch your spine up as if you had a pillow under it.
- Hips and thighs: Lie on your back, lock your knees and press your heels down into the surface you're resting on.
- Lower legs and feet: Curling the toes downward, try to touch the bottom of your feet with them. Then bend them the other way, toward your knees.

How do you feel now? Probably more relaxed than you've felt in a long time. You've just banished tension from your whole body. And now when you feel tension in just one muscle group, you can use what you've learned to work on that one part. I call it tension search and destroy.

Tips for Success

It took me a good 20 minutes to go through the above routine. And to tell you the truth, I ran into a couple of problems you might want to be on the lookout for. First, it's not easy to tense only one muscle group while leaving the rest of your body relaxed. I'd get as far as my stomach only to find my jaw stiffening up. But by rechecking for tension in muscle groups—and redoing them if necessary—I was eventually able to achieve precise body control. With a little practice (possibly even several PR sessions), you can do the same.

Second, concentrating during these exercises can be tough. The mind can be almost infuriating in its tendency to wander away from the business at hand. If you feel your attention slipping, stop. Try again later. Luckily, I found that with each fresh attempt, my concentration got better.

To enhance your power over stress, you may want to try progressive relaxation in conjunction with some other technique. Autogenic training and guided imagery are two ways to boost your ability to relax.

Soothing music can help, too. I've found bookstores to be a good source of relaxation tapes. You may want to look into tapes by two prominent stress-reduction experts: Emmett Miller, M.D., and Steven Halpern, Ph.D. Dr. Halpern's "Anti-Frantic" tapes, currently quite popular, are made up entirely of music specifically composed to induce relaxation and harmony. Dr. Miller produces a wide assortment of relaxation tapes, some incorporating a mixture of music, guided imagery and positive affirmation.

Jog Your Memory

Memory. People tend to think of it as the ability to dredge up the name of that mustached man they met in a Parisian pet shop 25 years ago. But in reality, we use our memory every minute of the day for everything we do. We use it every time we speak a word, drive a car, brush our teeth, or shop for groceries.

Given the importance of memory, it's hard to understand why we do so little to keep this important commodity from declining as we get older. Maybe it's because we don't think there's anything we can do about it. But in fact, the regeneration of a fading memory is well within most people's power.

"Many of the everyday lapses we experience are more the fault of our poor memory techniques than of any physical problem with the brain," says Robin West, Ph.D., University of Florida psychologist and author of *Memory Fitness over Forty.* "Given the use of good techniques, practice, and daily mental stimulation, there's no reason why you can't improve your memory substantially."

Keeping your memory in top form is similar to keeping your body in shape. But instead of brisk morning strolls, you need to turn the task of memorizing into a creative adventure that makes your mind work up a healthy sweat. Here's how to set up your own memory training program.

Attenn-shun!

Start by memorizing a little one-liner penned by English writer Samuel Johnson: "The art of memory is the art of attention." When we can't remember a piece of information, frequently it's because we never really paid enough attention to it in the first place. Since we didn't encode it firmly in our memory, it's no surprise that it's not there when we look for it.

Taking the attention theme one step further, in 1890, psychologist William James wrote, "Habit diminishes the conscious attention with which our acts are performed." To put this ponderous statement into everyday clothes, try to remember in detail the sign above the first gas station that you pass on the way to the grocery store or work. Don't feel bad if you can't. Even though you pass it every day, chances are you never really see it. "People commonly turn off their minds when they are performing habitual actions," says Dr. West. "When you are in an 'automatic pilot mode,' new information has no way of encoding itself in your mind."

The way to combat automatic-pilot syndrome is to practice the fine art of observation—consciously pay attention to details that make an object or circumstance unique. Dr. West suggests starting with a magazine photo of a person. Look at the photo, then close the magazine. List the features in the photo. What color were the eyes? What shape was the nose? What about hairstyle and clothing? Was there anything in the background? Having made a list, go back to the photo and study it for two details you missed. Then start again. Do this until you've managed to list every aspect down to the most minute.

Another way to practice observation during the day is to think of a common item that you see regularly. It could be a fountain pen, a building you walk by, or a tile floor. Before you actually come across the item again, ask yourself some questions about it. What is it made of? How many windows? What color? If you can't answer the questions immediately, take a moment when confronted by the object to look for the answers.

With practice, observation can become second nature. The way you look at things changes as you focus in on details. And the attention you pay to detail makes each object unique enough that it will stand out in your mind and be easily encoded into your memory.

Off Automatic Pilot

Now you can apply your new-found powers of observation to your behavior. How many times have you left the house only to wonder 10 minutes later if you locked the front door? "To overcome an automatic-pilot behavior like this, you need to either change the pattern of your action or find something concerning this routine action that is new and unusual," says Dr. West.

If you're right-handed, for example, you could lock the front door with your left hand. Or, as you lock the door, note the sound of the lawn mower coming from your neighbor's yard. Twenty minutes later, as you're driving along wondering whether you locked the front door, you'll remember the lawn mower and then remember that you locked the door while listening to that sound.

Making Things Meaningful

Memory and learning are not far apart, notes Dr. West. When we learn, we take random information and arrange it in a manner that has meaning to us.

As we concentrate and note specific details, they become encoded in our memory. But many things we wish to remember, such as lists of items, phone numbers, dates, and random facts, are difficult to organize into a cohesive whole because they have no order or inherent meaning. Rather than remembering one thing that naturally flows into another, we try to remember many different pieces of information that have no connection.

A better way—and the secret of most memory techniques—involves organizing those small pieces of material into larger groups, giving the items a context we can understand and making the information unique in our own minds.

"Many times, it's hard to draw a line of understanding between a word and its meaning," says Dr. West. "You might be hard put to remember that the medical prefix *blepharo-* refers to the eyelids, for example, because it provides no clues. But you can take the sound of the word and incorporate it into this sentence: "I'd blink if I saw a pharaoh." The sentence reminds you of the word and blink suggests eyelid."

To remember an address, such as 1225 Turner Street, you might say to yourself, "I turned my life around on Christmas," (12/25). Can't seem to remember that there are 5,280 feet in a mile? Think of "5 tomatoes": 5, 2(to), 8(mat), 0(oes).

Interactive Imagery

Here's a good memory technique to practice at the supermarket. Suppose you have six items you need to pick up. To use mental imagery, picture the six items in your mind. Maybe they'd be on a shelf or lined up at the checkout counter, but the six items would be inactive.

Interactive imagery goes one step further, in that you picture a sequence of action events that include the items you want to remember. That way, when you're at the store, you can just replay the image in your mind like a video. It may sound confusing, but let's give it a whirl using a typical grocery list: milk, bread, celery, pepper, apples, and cucumbers. Keep in mind that the more flamboyant the image, the better you'll remember it.

Walking through the woods, you come to the bank of a white river of milk. To make your journey easier, you decide to sail down the river and do so on a raft made of a large slice of bread. The long green steering oar you're using is actually an enormous celery stalk. The weather starts to turn bad, and soon dense flakes of black snow (pepper) and huge red hailstones (apples) begin to fall. Things go from bad to worse as your bread raft sails out to a milk sea where an enemy submarine is waiting. The sub fires and you see a cucumber torpedo heading straight for you.

Now close your eyes and try very hard to actually see yourself in the story. Once you have seen the image, try testing yourself and see if you remember all six items by replaying your mental video. Try again five days from now.

This technique can also be applied to other tasks, such as remembering names. "When I want people to remember my name," says Dr. West, "I have them picture a robin flying west. To connect the name to my person, I ask them to include my most memorable feature, long hair, in the image. The end result is a mental image of a robin flying west with long hair streaming behind it in the wind. When they see my long hair, it triggers the image that contains my name, Robin West."

If you are thinking that this is an awful lot of trouble just to remember a few things, note the other benefits that will accrue. "Storing information in a rich, elaborate form is the secret of sharp recall," says psychologist Endel Tulving, Ph.D., of the University of Toronto.

The process of making information rich and elaborate is also one of the finest ways to stimulate yourself intellectually. Your mind needs this stimulation to stay sharp just as your heart needs aerobic exercise to stay strong. And you may just find that tailoring information into sayings and images can be quite an entertaining way to stay in mental shape.

Finally, if you don't exercise your memory, you will begin to lose it. There's little doubt about that, experts agree. Most of the time, the process can be reversed, but why not start to recharge your memory now and enjoy it to the fullest?

Beyond Book Learning

Many of us remember (some with pride, some with loathing) the tests of IQ, or intelligence quotient, that we took back in grade school. As it turns out, the time-honored Stanford-

Binet IQ test, primarily a measurement of problem-solving speed and knowledge, is a fair predictor of scholastic success. But is this test a good indicator of success in the real world?

There are many psychologists who now feel that it's not. They're finding that intelligence consists of many more functions than those currently tested by Stanford-Binet—and that a few of those functions may be larger contributors to lifetime success than formal IQ. In other words, while you may not have had straight A's in school, you may still have the stuff that company presidents are made of.

"I would argue that intelligence is all the abilities that help us achieve our goals," says Jonathan Baron, Ph.D., professor of psychology at the University of Pennsylvania. "Problem-solving speed and knowledge are useful, but focusing solely on these aspects leaves out a great deal that's important to achieving goals successfully throughout life."

Rational thinking, as Dr. Baron calls it, is one very important kind of intelligence that is often overlooked. To understand the nature of rational thinking and why it is more relevant to your life in general, just compare a typical IQ-test question: "Complete this sequence: 3, 5, 9, 15," to a real-life problem: "How should you invest your life savings?"

The correct answer to the first question is 23. While life might be simpler if there were a single, correct response to the second question, it's obvious that there is no absolute right answer. Most of the problems we deal with in life are like the second question. "Should we have another child?" "Should I hire this person or that one?" How we answer questions that do not have absolute answers is where rational thinking comes into play.

The Elements of Rational Thinking

"I see rational thinking as being divided into two parts," says Dr. Baron. "The first part consists of a search in which we look for possible solutions, evidence, and goals. The second part is inference. Here we use the evidence to strengthen or weaken the possibilities with our goals in mind."

Let's run through a hypothetical situation and see how it all comes together. It's your Aunt Myra's birthday and you want to do something special for her. The possibilities might include throwing her a surprise party, taking her out to dinner at the most elegant restaurant in town, taking her to a heavy-metal rock concert, or buying her a nice gift. Evidence from past experiences tells you that she is embarrassed by undue attention (e.g., surprise parties), mistrusts any food prepared in a restaurant, and turns blue when rock music is played. Combining all this information from your search, you realize (inference) that a gift would best fulfill your goal of making Aunt Myra happy. It may not be the absolute right answer, but it is a good answer.

A Higher Level of Thought

Questions that require rational thinking are typically more akin to lifetime value judgments. They require a much higher level of complex and subtle reasoning, and a certain amount of impartiality. How would you answer this question, for example: "In general, do you think that capital punishment is necessary for our society?" "Your level of rational thinking would depend, in part, on how open-minded you are to the question," says Dr. Baron.

Many people develop an intuitive answer to this kind of question early in life and spend the rest of their lives defending that answer. They might look only at evidence that supports their side of the argument. But if you look at only 50 percent of the evidence on any question, you're denying yourself the possibility of achieving a higher-quality judgment. "It's rather like judging a man innocent after hearing only the evidence from the defending attorney," says Dr. Baron. "Rational thinking demands that you look at opposing evidence."

Learn to Think Better

We all may harbor the potential to be good rational thinkers, but we need a catalyst to develop this form of intelligence to the fullest.

"You can start out by taking a college-level course," suggests Dr. Baron. "Most classes require you to make some attempt at comparing conflicting views on a topic and forming a logical conclusion. You have the additional benefit of learning from your professor where you went wrong."

Or try to achieve mental flexibility in everyday surround-
ings. Read books that hold opposing views from your own and
try to understand why the author might be right. If you think
the author has some valid views, try to incorporate them into
your own framework and re-form your opinion.

Even getting into a good old-fashioned intellectual argument can help, but "only if you respect the other person's
opinions, answer them thoughtfully, and back up your argument with evidence," says Dr. Baron.

Here are a few well-chosen suggestions from Dr. Baron
that you may want to consider before you make your next
decision.

- Ask yourself if you may be avoiding thinking.
- Consider alternatives.
- Ask yourself how you would respond to the evidence if you
didn't care what was true.
- Remember that doing nothing is just as much a choice as
doing something.
- Don't decide on your final "best choice" before gathering all
the evidence.
- Understand that you can't make something best if it isn't.
- Be a detective, not a warrior.

Patient, Heal Thyself

Imagine, if you will, the brightest possible future for medicine. One in which even those chronic diseases most unrespon-
sive to treatment yield, finally, to a new medical paradigm. And
even better, imagine that this new approach teaches the body
to use its own natural defenses—and ultimately, eliminates the
use of harsh drugs and surgery to fight disease.

International researchers following in the footsteps of Ivan
Pavlov are working now to bring that future to reality. And if
they succeed, their work could forever change the face of
medicine.

You may recall that Pavlov rang a bell when lab animals were fed; later the sound of the bell alone was enough to make those animals salivate—despite the absence of food. Medical researchers soon realized that this was more than just a neat trick and designed experiments to see what other physical responses could be conditioned.

In 1982, for example, researchers at the University of Rochester gave mice lupus, a disease in which the body comes under attack by its own immune system. To combat the lupus, a powerful drug that suppresses the immune system was given to the mice—along with a drink of saccharin-sweetened water.

After this conditioning period, the drug treatment was stopped for some of the mice, and only the sweetened water was given. Astonishingly, the animals who got only the water fought off the effects of the lupus just as well as mice who continued to receive the drug. And no, there isn't anything special about saccharin—the researchers were careful to make sure that it didn't affect lupus by testing a separate set of mice who received only the sweetener and not the drug (*Annals of the New York Academy of Sciences*).

In similar experiments, Vithal Ghanta, Ph.D., associate professor of biology and microbiology in the neurosciences program at the University of Alabama at Birmingham, used the smell of camphor to control cancer in mice.

New Hope for the Future

Dr. Ghanta and her colleagues did their experiments with bone marrow cancer—a particularly deadly form of the disease. "There's generally not a lot you can do for patients that have this cancer—it's usually fatal," she says.

The researchers gave 50 mice injections of a drug that causes the body to produce more interferon. This in turn augments the natural killer-cell activity that fights that particular cancer (among other diseases). The researchers repeated this nine times, each time exposing the mice to the strong smell of camphor (mothballs) around the time of the injection. Then they induced bone-marrow cancer in the mice.

Finally, the mice were divided into three groups: One group continued to receive the drug, the second got no treatment, and the third continued to sniff camphor on a regular basis.

The mice who received the drug survived only a little longer than the group that got no treatment at all. The group that got only the camphor, however, did much better. Three out of ten went into remission. One later relapsed, but the other two survived to live out a normal life span (*Annals of the New York Academy of Sciences*).

"I'm not entirely satisfied with the results," says Dr. Ghanta. "After all, it's only a 20 percent success rate." She acknowledges, however, that previous results in defeating such cancers have not been very encouraging. By comparison, 20 percent seems like a promising figure.

A Safer Alternative

The camphor-treated animals' internal systems had been conditioned to mimic the effects of the drug. Why then, didn't some of the mice who continued to receive the drug treatment survive as well?

"The drugs used to combat cancer are extremely toxic," says Dr. Ghanta. "That's why we're pursuing the angle of conditioning—to get the benefits of the drug without the toxic side effects."

While this experiment exposed the mice to the drug/camphor combination nine times before trying the camphor alone, Dr. Ghanta has also attained good results after just one pairing of a drug and a conditioning stimulus (a strong taste, smell, sight, or sound that causes the body to "recall" the active treatment).

And the effects have been found to linger for quite a while. In other camphor studies by Dr. Ghanta, the benefits held firm for about ten subsequent exposures to the stimulus alone.

Of Mice and Men

"Obviously, our goal is to eventually use this treatment to reduce the toxic side effects of drugs and thus improve cancer survival in humans," says Dr. Ghanta. "But our work is still at a very early stage of development. Before we move on to humans, we want to improve the survival rates of the mice. We also need to know why it works.''

That understanding is necessary because many cancers can't be controlled by the type of body defenses these mice were conditioned to marshal. ''If we were to move directly to experiments with humans right now, we'd be limited to working with the cancers that respond well to interferon,'' she says. ''Unfortunately, interferon is only effective against a few types of cancer.

''But there's no reason to believe that the effects of conditioning are limited to any specific types of cancer,'' she adds. ''It's just that each type will probably require a different 'active' part of the therapy that does help fight that specific cancer.''

Human Evidence

''Actually, there have been studies that show conditioning to work very well in humans,'' says Novera H. Spector, Ph.D., health scientist and administrator in the Division of Fundamental Neurosciences at the National Institutes of Health.

Back in the 1960s, Russian scientists were able to both stimulate and depress people's immune systems through conditioning, he says. ''Some scientists feel that those studies need to be repeated before they can be taken seriously. But I've looked at the data carefully, and many of the experiments are very well done. They show conclusively that humans can be conditioned.''

Furthermore, he says, a study in which humans have been able to raise their own natural killer-cell production through conditioning is currently under way in Europe. The details will be available as soon as the study is completed.

Dr. Spector feels certain that the findings of those European researchers will clear the way for American human studies to begin. ''The evidence is now very good that conditioning will work in humans. In fact, I'm sure that it will work.''

By using this technique, he says, we may not only enhance the effectiveness of many drugs but actually avoid them entirely in some cases. ''The body, after all, is the ultimate medicine chest; it may supply what we need to fight a variety of diseases and chronic conditions. But first, we need to be able to teach ourselves to release those naturally occurring substances on command.''

A World of Cures

Research has already shown that a wide variety of responses can be conditioned. "Studies done in the 1960s showed that both body temperature and blood pressure can be conditioned," says Dr. Spector. "More recently, studies have shown that conditioning can stimulate the immune system to combat cancer, or depress it to fight autoimmune conditions like lupus." Although it hasn't been tested directly, researchers suspect that the same principle can be applied to fighting arthritis. It's even been shown that conditioning can reduce an allergic reaction.

"Just about any physiological reaction can be conditioned," says Dr. Spector. "All you have to do is figure out what response in the body can affect the disease in question, then design a conditioning situation that will 'call up' that response."

That's just what's been happening at the Army's Research Institute of Environmental Studies in Natick, Massachusetts. Researchers there conditioned people with Raynaud's syndrome—a painful condition that cuts circulation to the hands in cold weather—to overcome their problem without the traditional answer of drugs or surgery.

The study subjects entered a room where the temperature had been dropped to the freezing point and immediately placed their hands into a warm water bath for 10 minutes. This procedure was repeated 54 times over six weeks. When the people were later exposed to cold, their fingers were able to stay almost 7 degrees warmer than before the treatment. They also reported less pain during subsequent attacks. Their bodies had been conditioned to dilate the blood vessels in their hands, rather than constrict them, in response to cold.

"The medical applications of what we've learned are obviously of vast importance," says Dr. Spector. "They offer exciting new prospects both in preventive medicine and in the treatment of many diseases. The doors are just being opened and the possibilities are endless.''

Body-Care Updates

Fighting Back against Backache

Blame it all on progress. You didn't hear Cro-Magnon man complaining about his aching back. Before some now-forgotten inventor threw some rocks together and designed the first chair, people either squatted or lay down when they needed to take a load off their feet. Both activities put far less pressure on the spine than sitting.

No wonder back pain is a problem for an estimated eight out of ten people: We sit for most of our 16 waking hours every day. Worse, a lot of us slouch in our chairs or sit hunched over work at a desk for long stretches of time.

A Simple Solution

There's a dramatically simple solution to much of this needless misery caused by too much chair time, says Phil Dunphy, exercise physiologist and physical therapist.

"Give yourself regular breaks from sitting," he advises. "If you sit all day, just stand up for 5 minutes every hour, and I guarantee your back will feel better. Stand when you talk on the phone, or take a short break and walk around at regular intervals while you're at work."

And what about those killer car trips that can leave you feeling about as limber as the Tin Man?

"You can avoid that back-killing posture by tilting your rearview mirror up a bit," Dunphy says. "You should have to sit up perfectly straight to see the cars behind you. If you can't see the cars, you know you're slumping and you're reminded to sit up.''

In short, the key to ending backache is to get more extension into your life. You want less flexion—less sitting all curled up and stooped over. Think about what happens when you yawn—your whole body straightens up and extends naturally. It feels good because there's less stress on your spine in that position.

Test Your Flexibility

Dunphy recommends an easy extension test to see how flexible your back is: Simply lie face-down on the floor. If your back hurts in that position, you could use some more flexibility.

The best way to correct that is to stand up straight, but that's not always as easy as it sounds. Dunphy suggests that you start a walking program as a way of getting used to standing up straight again. "But you have to walk correctly," he warns. "A lot of people are all bent over when they walk. Stand up with your back against a wall. Now get out and walk exactly like that.

"It's also important to keep your head level when you walk," says Dunphy. "If you do that, you're automatically in the extension posture that's good for your back."

You can also fight back pain through exercise. "The key to a pain-free back is muscles strong enough to keep the spine in proper alignment," says California physical therapist Gregory Johnson.

But exercise can do more than just strengthen back muscles, adds Georgia physical therapist Russel Gill. "If done properly, exercises give an internal massage to tense muscles of the back. The right activities subject the spine to gentle rotations and compressions."

Maintain a Correct Position

The right activity is key, emphasizes Dunphy. And at the core of right activity is maintaining the correct position while you're working out.

With that in mind, here's his advice on the best and worst workouts for a bad back.

Best

Nordic ski machine. These machines give you a good overall workout and allow you to stand the entire time. "You get progressive resistance, a great aerobic workout, and the upper- and lower-body development you need to take the strain off your back when you do things that require some strength," says Dunphy. "If you're not used to working out, just do 5 minutes to start and work up gradually until you can go for 30 or 40 minutes."

Walking. With the right posture, Dunphy says, this is the perfect exercise. Start slow and work up to 30 or 40 minutes, three or four times a week. A treadmill is a good alternative when the weather turns nasty.

Not Bad

Cycling. If you ride a bike, he says, bring the handlebars all the way up and move the seat up—not all the way up but higher than you normally would. That way you're not all slumped over.

Rowing machine. It's okay, but only if you can sit up straight on your machine, notes Dunphy. Many machines are designed strictly for an upper-body workout and can't be adjusted to keep your back from curling. If you can, try a few out in the store before deciding which one to buy.

Swimming. A great exercise for your back if you've got good form, Dunphy says. That means a straight-leg kick that keeps you flat in the water. If you're sinking all the time, you're in a flex position that's bad for your back.

Weight training. Lifting weights can really help you to stand up straight by giving you the upper- and lower-body development that takes the strain off your back. Again, though, the key is proper form. And, as Dunphy points out, good form isn't easy to come by. Unless you have a good instructor to help you learn the proper techniques, you could be running the risk of exacerbating your back problem with weights.

Worst

Running. It's not wise to take up running if you have back problems. "In moderation it would be fine, but I've never seen anyone who didn't take it too far, push too hard," says Dunphy.

Tennis and racquetball. Don't even think about these if you have a bad back. They're both great aerobic exercises, he says, but you're stooped over the whole time you're playing.

Seven Common Causes of Contact Allergy

The field of allergy is a bit oddly divided. If your symptoms are provoked by an allergy to foods or inhalants (like dust or pollen), your best choice among physicians is an allergist.

But if your allergy problem only occurs when you come in contact with a specific substance, such as jewelry or a cosmetic component, you need the help of a dermatologist.

The patients who have chosen to see Leonard Grayson, M.D., get both. One of the very few American physicians to be board-certified in both allergy and dermatology, Dr. Grayson has a unique opportunity to observe—and treat—pretty much all the various problems that allergy can cause.

For several years now, Dr. Grayson has been spreading his knowledge of contact allergy among traditional allergists. Teaming up with fellow dermatologist Lucia Fischer-Papp, M.D., he offers an extremely popular workshop on contact allergy diagnosis and treatment at major allergy conferences.

Here are just a few of the things reported at the recent conference of the American Academy of Allergy and Immunology in Anaheim, California.

Nix Rub-On Antihistamines • "Topical lotions that contain antihistamines (like Caladryl) are so drying that they just don't relieve the itching and discomfort of contact allergy reactions.

And they're extremely sensitizing in themselves, meaning that they're a known cause of frequent contact allergy problems.

"People should just stick to good old calamine lotion—especially for problems like poison ivy where the skin can become broken and greatly irritated."

Watch Drug-Patch Warnings • "Transdermal patches, which deliver medication slowly over a period of weeks, are causing contact allergy reactions in a number of people. If people are using these patches, say for blood pressure control, they should contact their doctor if any kind of a rash appears."

Prevent Nail Polish Problems • "Nail polish doesn't cause problems after it's dry, but while it's wet, it can be a common source of contact allergy reactions—especially if you touch your eyes or any area of your face while your nails are still wet.

"Use a hair dryer for about 15 or 20 minutes to dry your nails right after you put on the polish, and you won't have any problems."

You *Can* Wear Your Watch • "If you're having contact allergy problems where the back of your watch meets your skin, it's probably a reaction to one of the metals used to make that portion of the watch, most likely nickel.

"You can get a product called Clear Seal at a hardware store or a five-and-dime and simply paint the back of the watch with it. That will make a protective barrier, and you'll be able to wear the watch without any problems. But it has to be repeated every few days."

Prevent Piercing Problems • "The easiest way to avoid developing an allergy to metals like nickel is to make sure that plastic posts are used when you have your ears pierced.

"If you already have the allergy and want to wear your favorite earrings on a special occasion, you can try putting a steroid cream right on the posts before you put them in your ears. But you shouldn't wear the earrings too often; it's for special occasions only."

Identify an Underarm Rash • "A rash in the area of the armpit is generally one of two things. If the rash is actually in the armpit itself, it's almost always a reaction to the deodorant that you're using.

"Simply changing brands may help, but if it doesn't, you have to get patch tested to see exactly what it is in the deodorant that you're reacting to. Then your dermatologist can help you find a brand that doesn't contain that substance. Or you can just use baking soda.

"But if the rash is around the outside of the armpit, it's likely to be a reaction caused by the formaldehyde present in all permanent-press clothing.

"Contact allergy caused by the formaldehyde in this type of fabric is fairly common, especially when the clothing is tight and the person perspires heavily. Loose-fitting clothes are much less likely to cause problems. Really hot and humid weather makes it worse.

"To avoid it entirely you'd have to shop for clothes that wrinkle easily! Some people have found that they can wear clothes that contain formaldehyde despite their allergy if they wear undergarments that are formaldehyde free."

Be Wary of "Temporary" Hair Dye • "As many people know, the chemical PPD, found in almost every permanent hair dye, can cause severe contact allergy reactions. As an alternative, some people have tried using the temporary, six-week, 'hair rinse' dyes.

"Unfortunately, these dyes also contain PPD and are every bit as sensitizing as the permanent ones. They are not safe for people who are allergic to PPD.

"People who are allergic to such dyes can use pure henna safely. They can also use peroxide, and they won't experience an allergic reaction to lead acetate dyes, although some people may not want to use products that contain lead on their skin.

"Another alternative is to find a cooperative hair stylist who will use the 'double-hood' tinting technique. This involves covering the person's head with a specially designed hood that completely covers the scalp yet allows the hair to be pulled through numerous little holes so that it can be treated."

Update on TMJ

By Andrew Kaplan, D.M.D.

Like many patients on their first visit, Joy Forrester was in evident pain. "I've had headaches all my life," she told me, "but nothing like this." During the past month she had become more and more incapacitated. Sometimes the pain seemed to radiate outward from behind her eyes and into her cheeks. Sometimes it shot upward from her temples to the top of her head. Lately pain and ringing had developed in her ears as well.

At first she thought her allergies were acting up and inflaming her sinuses. "Allergic to everything I breathe," she received year-round shots and a variety of drugs to keep her symptoms under control. So she went first to her allergist, who prescribed a powerful steroid medication to reduce inflammation. It didn't work. Rather, as steroids often do, it irritated her digestive tract and quickly had to be abandoned. Then began a procession of visits to several other baffled physicians, while the pain grew worse.

She saw a neurologist, a gynecologist, an internist, an ear, nose and throat specialist (otolaryngologist), and another allergist. Severe chronic headaches are among the most difficult of all symptoms to treat successfully, since they can have so many different causes. All these physicians could do for her was eliminate one possible diagnosis after another.

Finally, after performing the usual tests and hearing her history, the second allergist she consulted concluded that her problem wasn't an allergy. "In fact," he told her, "just about all the usual reasons for your headaches appear to have been considered. But there is one other possibility."

"What's that?"

"You may be suffering from a TMJ disorder." She had never heard of it. "Let me show you what I mean."

Tracing Pain to the Jaw

The allergist placed his fingertips on the sides of her face, just in front of her ears, and pressed lightly. "I almost passed out from the pain," she reported. The doctor explained that the tender areas were in the joints that connected her lower jaw to her skull: the temporomandibular joints, or TMJs. "TMJ disorders aren't usually treated by physicians," he said. "They're treated by dentists."

And that's how Joy Forrester eventually came to my office. My colleagues and I see several hundred TMJ patients each year. Many of them have never heard of the TMJ, much less TMJ disorders.

Their main complaint is pain, pain that is often persistent, agonizing, and debilitating. The pain may occasionally subside, giving the sufferer the illusion that it is gone for good, only to reappear, often worse than ever, days, weeks or months later. It may vary during the day: For some it is worse in the morning, for others, in the afternoon or evening. For some it may be relentless and unremitting, all day and every day. The emotional suffering is perhaps even worse than the physical pain. As they continue to suffer, these patients become absorbed in their pain: It takes over their lives. Many become unable to work or to cope with the ordinary tasks of day-to-day living.

One patient admitted to me in mortification that she had virtually handed over her small children to the care of a neighbor. She just couldn't manage her household and her pain at the same time.

The suffering is often reinforced by frustrating medical experiences. Many physicians either give up or prescribe treatment that turns out to be ineffective. Frequently, patients are urged to seek psychiatric help in the mistaken belief that their problems are "all in their heads."

TMJ-disorder pain is deceptive. It baffles many health professionals, and it certainly baffles the unfortunate patients. It doesn't have to be located in or near the joint at all. Joy Forrester's headaches are typical, but there are many other examples.

The Root of a Mysterious Toothache

For instance, a middle-aged woman made five visits to the Mount Sinai dental clinic complaining of a persistent ache in one of her molars. But there was nothing wrong with the tooth that anyone could find—no decay, no abscess, no painful sensitivity to tapping, heat, or cold. The dental residents were prepared to start root-canal treatment in hope that it would relieve her pain, but one of them asked me to take a look first.

I found a small, hard knot of muscle in the middle of the woman's cheek. I asked the resident for the lidocaine syringe with which he was about to anesthetize the tooth. I injected a small amount of anesthetic into the knot. In less than a minute, a look of astonishment came over the woman's face. "The pain is gone," she said. "This is the first time in two months that tooth hasn't hurt!"

The tooth wasn't the source of her pain at all. The pain was referred to the tooth from the area of constricted muscle. And the muscle constriction was in turn caused by a TMJ disorder. Eventually we were able to relieve all her problems.

Another typical example: A young woman was referred to the clinic by an ear, nose, and throat specialist. She had gone to him with a severe earache, but he could find no sign of infection or any other problem with her ear. Fortunately he was familiar with TMJ disorders and their capacity for producing symptoms elsewhere, so he sent her to us. We were not surprised to find that she had a nervous habit of grinding her teeth and that her jaw made a noticeable clicking sound when she opened and closed it. Further examination confirmed a TMJ disorder. Treating it soon got rid of her earache.

A Summary of Self-Help

Treating TMJ disorders is mainly a job for professionals: dentists, physical therapists, psychologists, surgeons, and so forth. Nonetheless, there are several things that you can do for yourself if you have a TMJ disorder, or think you may have one, or want to avoid getting one.

Check Your Symptoms • Do-it-yourself diagnosis is unwise and sometimes dangerous. This is especially true of TMJ disorders—the "painful pretenders." Even so, certain characteristic symptoms may make it wise for you to ask your physician or dentist about consulting a TMJ practitioner.

Among them:

- Headaches, often severe and recurrent. They tend to occur more commonly on one side than on both and in areas around the eyes, cheeks and temples, but they can also occur at the top or base of the skull.
- Toothaches that cannot be traced to decay, nerve death, or inflammation.
- Burning or tingling sensations, especially in the tongue but sometimes in the mouth or throat.
- Earaches or "stuffed" sensations in the ears, sometimes accompanied by dizziness or by ringing or rushing noises.
- Neckaches, shoulder aches or backaches, sometimes accompanied by numbness in the arms or hands.
- Tenderness and swelling, particularly in the sides of the face.
- Clicking or popping noises when opening the jaw, closing it, or both.
- Inability to open the mouth freely, either because of pain or because some impediment seems to "lock" the jaw at a certain point. If the problem occurs on one side only, the jaw may not open straight but slide off to one side.

Use Medications Wisely • Many of the medications and other procedures used to treat TMJ disorders must be administered by professionals. But you can obtain certain effective pain relievers over the counter.

Medications should be used sparingly and not over a long period. Otherwise they tend to hide the disorder rather than cure it. But I see no harm in them when used to relieve acute pain, and some of them need no prescription.

Aspirin is a very effective analgesic (painkiller), with coated forms for those with sensitive stomachs. Aspirin also helps reduce inflammation in muscle and joint tissues.

Most anti-inflammatory medications require a prescription, but ibuprofen is available over the counter in very mild form. Taken as instructed, it may relieve pain, but it won't be strong enough to control inflammation. And it isn't safe for you to take larger doses without professional supervision.

Salves and sprays containing local anesthetics can give temporary relief to sore muscles like the masseter and temporalis. Be careful to keep them away from your eyes.

Avoid Caffeine • This is one way to control the pain of inflammation. Caffeine stimulates the central nervous system, increases muscle tension, and increases sensitivity to pain. The strongest source is coffee, but tea, chocolate, and cola drinks also contain caffeine.

Limit Jaw Movement • Open your jaws only as far as you can without feeling pain, and avoid wide opening. If you feel a yawn coming, restrict it by pressing a fist under your chin.

Eat a Soft Diet • You don't have to switch entirely to liquids and baby food. But avoid foods like raw vegetables, nuts, hard rolls, and chewy meat such as steak. Also avoid chewing gum. For main dishes, use pasta and noodles or casseroles and hashes made with chopped or minced meat, fish, or eggs. Substitute cooked vegetables and fruits for raw ones.

Apply Heat and Cold • These are old but effective remedies for relieving pain and reducing inflammation. Some patients respond better to one than the other, and some are helped most by the use of the two in succession.

Methods of heat application include the moist compress, a towel or other absorbent fabric soaked in hot water. A hot water bottle applied over the compress will keep it warm longer.

Also available are professional devices such as the Hydrocolator, available at hospital-supply stores and some drugstores. It contains a fluid-filled plastic pouch that is inserted into a fabric wrapper held in place with Velcro fasteners.

The simplest way to apply cold is in the form of ice. I recommend sealing it in a plastic bag, which is then wrapped in a dry cloth. You can also use a ready-made cold pack, which remains flexible even when chilled below the freezing temperature of water. A "snap pack" doesn't even have to be chilled.

Striking it on a hard surface sets off a chemical reaction that makes it lose heat quickly.

A caution: Don't apply ice for more than about 20 minutes in any hour or you can damage your skin.

Correct Bad Posture • Physical therapists often instruct TMJ patients in special exercises designed to give greater flexibility to the muscles of the head and neck. Just as important are efforts to correct bad posture and other physical habits that contribute to TMJ disorders and interfere with recovery. These include:

• The forward-positioned head with the head thrust forward and the chin tilted up. Sometimes called "bird-watcher's posture," this is the most harmful of postural faults. The weight of your head puts undesirable pressure on the neck and back muscles and also strains the TMJs themselves.
• An exaggerated military posture, with the chest thrust forward and the chin up, is almost as harmful as a forward slump. Your chest and shoulders should be in a relaxed position, with your head balanced at the top of your neck and your chin tucked in.

You can assure good standing posture by using the natural weight distribution of your body. Instead of standing with your weight concentrated over your heels, rock forward slightly so your weight is mainly on the balls of your feet. As the weight of your lower body shifts forward, your head and shoulders will naturally settle back to serve as a balancing counterweight.

Many chairs don't support the middle and lower back but instead encourage slumping. You can insert a small cushion between your back and the chair to provide the missing support.

It also helps not to sit cross-legged or to sit for a long time in one position without a break.

When you drive, make sure the seat isn't too far back or too low in relationship to the dashboard so that you have to lean forward to see the road. If the seat won't adjust sufficiently, extra cushions behind or under you can sometimes make up the difference.

When you lie down, the worst fault is lying on your stomach with your head twisted to one side. Almost as bad is lying on your back with your head propped up at a sharp angle for reading or watching television.

The healthiest and most restful lying position is on the side, with a pillow thick enough to support the head and neck horizontally, and the arms and legs loosely flexed.

Other positions and habits to avoid:

• Cradling the telephone between shoulder and chin.
• Propping the chin on one or both hands for extended periods.
• Reaching high overhead for burdens.
• Painting, hammering, or doing other work on high walls or ceilings.
• Carrying a heavy shoulder bag with the strap on the same shoulder for an extended period.
• Wearing high-heeled boots or shoes.

Often the most effective form of posture reeducation is simply increased awareness. Once you're aware of the problem, it is usually not difficult to correct. At first, you may only correct the unhealthy habit when you're thinking about it, but gradually this conscious correction will become translated into a new, healthy habit.

Break the Teeth-Clenching Habit • Clenching or grinding teeth is widely believed to be a major cause of TMJ disorders. You can fight the habit by trying to keep your mouth in what we call the "healthy resting position."

Open your jaw slightly, so the upper and lower teeth are separated. Rest your tongue lightly against the roof of your mouth without pressing against the front teeth. Keep your lips shut so that you breathe through your nose. With practice, this position may itself become a habit, reducing the urge to clench or grind.

Retrain Your Body's Whole Response to Stress • To overcome clenching and grinding, it is often necessary to retrain your body's whole response to stress.

There are many forms of professional stress therapy, ranging from psychotherapy to biofeedback. But there are a
few simple physical and mental exercises that you can try on
your own.

• Deep-breathing exercises. Inhale slowly and deeply, counting to five at 1-second intervals. Between counts, think of a
single word (such as calm or peace) to help free your mind of
distracting or stressful thoughts. Hold your breath for 1 second, then exhale slowly, counting backward from five to one,
and silently repeat your chosen word. At the same time, let
your chest and stomach muscles relax, and drop your shoulders. Repeat this cycle three times.
• Progressive relaxation exercises. Tense and then relax
groups of related muscles in progression, over the whole body.
There is no set order, but you might start with the hands
(making a fist), proceed to the feet (curling the toes), and end at
the head (wrinkling the forehead). Tensing the muscles before
relaxing them seems to produce a greater degree of relaxation
than just trying to relax them.
• Guided imagery. This technique induces relaxation by calling up to "the mind's eye" a series of soothing sensory images.
You develop a mental image of a pleasant, tranquil experience
to which you consciously guide your attention. At first this
method is used just for training, to reduce emotional tension.
But, like breathing exercise or progressive relaxation, it eventually becomes habitual and can be used to provide relief in
stressful life situations.

Cutting Your Chances of a TMJ Disorder

The exact causes of TMJ disorders are still not completely
understood, so it is impossible to say that doing certain things,
or not doing others, will surely keep you from getting it. Nonetheless, evidence points to two conditions that at least predispose people to TMJ problems. One is malocclusion; the
other is clenching and grinding the teeth.

I have already described techniques to overcome clenching and grinding. The best defense against malocclusion is to
take care of your teeth. A common cause of malocclusion is

tooth loss as a result of poor care of the teeth and gums. Yet modern techniques make it likely—not just possible—that you can retain your natural teeth in good working order for your whole life.

Follow your dentist's advice. Brush regularly, and use dental floss and gum stimulators. Have your teeth checked and professionally cleaned twice a year, and don't let tooth decay or gum inflammation go untreated.

A question may have occurred to you: If restorative dentistry and orthodontics are so useful in stabilizing TMJ treatment, should they be used to prevent TMJ disorders? Based on present knowledge, the answer is: not for that reason alone. True, these techniques can and do remedy malocclusion, and malocclusion is implicated in TMJ disorders. But many people

---

SELF-TESTS FOR TMJ TROUBLE

To obtain evidence of a possible TMJ disorder, you can perform these simple self-tests.

1. Place the first two fingertips of each hand directly in front of each ear. The TMJs are directly underneath your fingers, and you should be able to feel their movement as you open and close your mouth. If even the light pressure of your fingertips causes pain on one or both sides, joint inflammation is a possibility.

2. Holding your hands near the sides of your face, tip them backward so the fingertips are pointing toward your ears. Place all four fingertips against the lower jaw on each side, with the index finger near the angle of the jaw. As you open and close you can feel the thick masseter muscles that extend diagonally from the angle to the cheekbone. Pain suggests the presence of myofascial pain dysfunction (MPD) resulting from muscle fatigue.

3. Press your fingers lightly against your temples above and in front of your ears. Open and close your mouth. If you feel pain, one or both of the fan-shaped temporalis muscles may be fatigued and sore.

If any of these self-tests causes discomfort, see your dentist for a professional diagnosis.

with even severe malocclusion never experience TMJ disorders. Also, some people with sound teeth and a good bite nonetheless develop these problems.

There are plenty of good reasons to undertake restorative dentistry or orthodontics. Appearance is one; another is a comfortable and efficient bite. But the evidence doesn't justify either procedure as a way to head off TMJ disorders.

Finally, there is one other, indisputable cause of temporomandibular-joint disorders, or at least a triggering circumstance: physical injury to the jaw. This usually results from accidents, especially auto accidents. So one of the things you can do to avoid TMJ disorders—and many other problems as well—is follow safety procedures at home and drive safely and defensively on the road.

How to Have Smooth, Supple Skin

Your skin is your body's first line of defense against a world teeming with chemicals, bacteria, and fungi. The system is just about flawless, until you allow its moisture balance to be upset.

"Skin that's constantly dry or cracked, and opens up easily, is more vulnerable to bacterial invasion," says Wilma Bergfeld, M.D., head of clinical dermatology research at the Cleveland Clinic Foundation. "The same is true of skin that's bloated with fluids. But informed use of moisturizers can help prevent such breaches of your body's defenses—and thus head off a lot of potential skin problems."

Skin Savvy

Knowing your skin type gets you off to a good start, because moisturizers are usually formulated for one of the three major skin types: dry, oily, or sensitive.

But even when you type-match your skin to a moisturizer, there are no guarantees. The variations in both cosmetic ingredients and your body's natural oils ensure that moisturizers work differently on everyone—even those with the same skin type. If a moisturizer keeps your skin supple without any negative side effects, you've got a winner.

A loser, when used repeatedly, can block pores and lead to blemishes. There's a way to reduce the chances of this happening, though. "Most of the larger cosmetic companies test their products to make them as noncomedogenic [not acne-causing] as possible," says Dr. Bergfeld. "If you routinely have trouble with blackheads or acne, I'd recommend that you select a moisturizer that states that it's been tested and found to be noncomedogenic." You could still be the 1 person in 10,000 who reacts to the product with blemishes, but at least the odds are in your favor.

Be on the lookout for perfumes and preservatives in moisturizers (and other cosmetics and soaps) that might cause you to develop contact dermatitis. "Many people come in complaining of dry, itchy facial skin. But when I examine them, they actually have contact dermatitis," Dr. Bergfeld says. It's a condition that scales (like dandruff) and may burn, sting, or itch. The best way to prevent this reaction is to have your dermatologist test you to determine which ingredient causes the problem, and then avoid it.

Remember to think twice about all the above considerations—once for your face and once for the rest of your body. Your facial skin may require one moisturizing formula, and the rest of your skin another. The skin on your face is more sensitive than elsewhere and may even be a different skin type.

"Eye-Deal"

Be careful what moisturizer you use around your eyes, because skin there is thinner. Anything that causes a reaction on the skin of your face will instigate a reaction four times greater around your eyes.

"It may be fine to use your moisturizer as an eye cream if it's an emollient only, with no active ingredient that claims to change the physiology of your skin (such as, 'Gets rid of wrinkles')," Dr. Bergfeld says. "But if your daily moisturizer claims to change your skin, consider using a separate eye cream.

"If you want it to double as an eye cream, use it elsewhere on your face for at least a month. Only if there have been no adverse reactions should you try it around your eyes."

A moisturizer formulated specifically for use around the eyes usually has a light texture that doesn't overwhelm the delicate skin in this area. Apply anything in this delicate area with a light hand. Use your ring finger and a patting motion to apply nourishment or makeup around the eyes.

A Balancing Act

Moisturizing is also tricky where there are skin folds, such as between your toes—places where you perspire more. Even without moisturizers these spots are susceptible to being over-hydrated—retaining too much fluid—a problem you rarely encounter on the face. Overhydration is frequently compounded by clothing or shoes that don't allow the sweat to evaporate.

"If you apply a moisturizer to wet skin, there's no chance of evaporation from the skin's surface. All the moisture that's generated is held there," explains Dr. Bergfeld.

"Athlete's foot is a good example of a problem that can be made worse by overhydration," she says. "When it's warm and moist between your toes, there's a warm 'garden' environment in which the fungus can flourish. Moisturizers may then provide the nutrients for that fungus to feed upon, especially if the product is old and the preservative in the oil is no longer working. If you have a fungal infection, you want to eliminate these ideal conditions. Keep the skin around your toes clean and dry and don't use a moisturizer there until the condition has disappeared."

So the general rule is avoid moisturizing in skin-fold areas unless they feel especially dry.

Applying It Smart

Before applying any moisturizer, ask yourself, "Is it fresh?"

"The shelf life of creams and lotions, as for all cosmetics, is a maximum of one to two years," says Dr. Bergfeld. "After that, the ingredients no longer have an agent that protects them against bacterial and fungal invasion. It's especially important to use fresh products around your eyes. We see a lot of problems with contaminated products getting into the eye, which is similar to putting a contaminated product in a cut."

When you apply a facial moisturizer, gently rub it on to relax underlying muscles, massaging for 10 seconds. The massage won't help get rid of wrinkles, but if it feels good, it may help ease stress lines a bit.

If your body skin is susceptible to pimples or other blemishes, try applying moisturizers in the direction of your hair follicles. Applying against the follicles makes them more likely to set up in the pores and cause problems.

If you have a skin infection, consult your dermatologist before applying any moisturizer. If a moisturizer stings, tingles, or itches when you put it on, you should probably avoid it. If it produces a rash, you'd better see a dermatologist to determine what caused it. It may be only one ingredient out of the ten that are in the product, but that one ingredient may be in many other products that you can avoid.

What to Do When You Overdo Fitness Fun

When outdoor workout weather finally comes each year, do you decide that this year you're going to exercise your body until it stops embarrassing you at the beach? Are you determined to hit the courts, the pools, the diamonds, the country trails? Are you sure you're going to love it? Of course. And are you going to hurt yourself? Yes. Sooner or later, you're bound to pay a small price for fitness fun—get a blister, a callus, a sprain, a backache, a cramp, a rash, a bruise, or something you least expect. So here's a guide to help you minimize all this and self-treat the hurts when they happen.

It lists specific ailments you're likely to encounter in your workouts. And it gives you current prevention and treatment advice from prominent experts.

A word to the wise-but-forgetful: The best guide to avoiding exercise injuries is still common sense. Before jumping into a sport or exercise program, check with your doctor to be sure you're in good enough shape to handle it. Take some time to prepare for your favorite sports by mastering proper form and by strengthening the parts of your body your activities tend to stress. Warm up gradually. Have access to a first-aid kit. And, especially in warm weather, drink plenty of cool water to fend off dehydration.

Backache

Sudden bending and twisting can put tremendous stress on your back, especially if your supporting abdominal and spinal muscles are weak initially. In general, the three keys to preventing back injuries are correct form, properly fitted equipment, and flexibility and strengthening exercises.

Cycling and swimming may encourage you to arch your spine too much, adding pressure to the lower back that can cause back pain. Cyclists who lean over the handlebars and have to arch their necks to see are most at risk.

James C. Puffer, M.D., head physician of the Summer Olympic Team says, "A crucial element in preventing back pain in cyclists is making sure their seat and handlebar height is appropriate." Adds Morris Mellion, M.D., chairman of the American Academy of Family Physicians' task force on sports medicine and committee on health education, "Your best bet is to go to a cycling shop that caters to racers and have the seat and handlebars adjusted."

Dr. Mellion says that the two main causes of back pain in swimmers are overuse—going from doing a little to doing a lot too fast—and incorrect form. He recommends varying your strokes to avoid overuse if you're prone to back pain. Any stroke is fine in moderation, although the whip kick (or frog kick) used in the breaststroke puts a lot of pressure on your lower back. Dr. Mellion also recommends having a swimming coach review your strokes with you. "Swimming lessons aren't just for kids," he says. "Adults ought to take lessons even if they're pretty good swimmers. Back pain among recreational swimmers is often better remedied by coaching than by medicine."

Golf and tennis players have to twist for powerful strokes. Almost every shot on a golf course involves torque from trunk rotation and can cause injury. Practicing on a driving range can put your back through the equivalent of 36 to 72 holes of golf in one hour. Golfers who weight their clubs are putting themselves at even higher risk of back injury. Like driving practice, tennis-serving practice twists the spine too quickly. Dr. Puffer advises both golfers and tennis players to take some lessons with a pro to make sure they're using correct form.

"Remember, though," he says, "in all sports you have to stop before you get too tired. Pushing yourself past the point of fatigue can strain your back as badly as incorrect form can. And your best protection against back pain is an exercise program aimed at strengthening the abdominal muscles, and stretching the hamstrings and lower back muscles. Keeping your weight down helps, too."

If you've managed to strain your back, you can ease the pain by applying ice and taking aspirin or acetaminophen until you get to a doctor for a complete evaluation.

"Bikini Bottom"

Wearing a swimsuit all day can cause "bikini bottom" (occlusive folliculitis), marked by annoying, pimplelike blisters all over the buttocks. When your skin soaks too long, explains Dr. Mellion, the tissue becomes vulnerable to infection. The bacteria normally present on your skin can cause boils, cysts, and acne when they penetrate the skin's protective outer layer.

Both Dr. Puffer and Dr. Mellion advise changing your bathing suit and drying off between swims. If it's already too late for that advice, your doctor may recommend a topical antibiotic acne preparation to heal your bumpy bottom.

Blisters

Blisters are the body's protest against too much friction. Once blisters form, don't let them tear. The best treatment is to protect them and let the fluid be reabsorbed. Dr. Puffer, who is also the chief of the Division of Family Medicine at UCLA, suggests using precut doughnut-shaped bandages (available at drugstores) to surround the blistered area with a cushioned surface.

If the blister is likely to break, try to drain it yourself, says Dr. Puffer. First clean it thoroughly with soap and water. Then, using a needle that you've sterilized in a flame, puncture the blister's edge. Press it gently with a sterile pad until all the fluid has drained out, then cover the blister with gauze. If the blister has already broken, clean the area gently with soap and water and cover with a sterile pad. Check frequently for signs of infection (like bright redness or pus), and see a doctor promptly if you find any.

Your best antiblister measure for feet is to wear shoes and socks that won't slip around on your skin. One way to ensure this no-slip wear is to double your socks, says Dr. Mellion. He suggests that you wear an inner sock made of a fabric that wicks perspiration away from your feet. (Wool or polypropylene are better than cotton.) And wear an outer sock (of medium thickness for tennis, heavier for hiking).

Buying shoes designed specifically for your sport can help if you make sure the shoe really fits. Allow enough room for your toes to move around, since your feet may swell considerably when you run or walk a lot.

When you buy golf clubs or any kind of rackets, don't assume that the grip that feels good corresponds to the proper size for you. Go to a reputable athletic or pro shop where they will take specific measurements to ensure the grips are properly sized for your hands. Dr. Puffer recommends wearing a glove on your racket hand to help minimize friction. Dr. Mellion adds that you can condition your playing hand to prevent blisters. "On your first few times out, don't start playing four times a week," he cautions. "Build up slowly from once or twice a week so your hands toughen gradually."

Calluses

A little toughening on your hands and feet is beneficial, protecting you from repeated friction. But when calluses begin to cause discomfort, it's probably time to see a doctor.

Those toughened patches of skin are often caused by friction from poorly fitted shoes or bad racket or golf-club grip. Severe callusing on your feet can also indicate some structural problem in your feet or spine. Your doctor may recommend arch supports or special pads. People with plantar warts (warts on the bottoms of their feet) often get calluses around them. Scars from cuts may also form calluses on your feet. Calluses can even form on your fingers when your racket, club, or bat rubs against a ring you're wearing.

"Soften foot calluses by soaking them for several minutes in warm water," says Dr. Puffer. "If you like, add a softening agent, such as foot soap. Next, wash the affected area with soap and water and dry it thoroughly. Then, using a pumice stone or callus file, gently scrape the surface to remove the top layer of toughened skin. Apply an adhesive-backed felt callus pad or doughnut so it surrounds but doesn't directly touch the tough area. The pad can help keep pressure off the damaged area to allow the skin to heal."

See a doctor if your calluses start to hurt or form an abnormal-looking growth. Dr. Puffer advises the same preventive measures for calluses as for blisters on page 285.

Eye Redness

Swimmers who prefer lakes and oceans often complain that chlorinated pools make their eyes red. Actually, says Dr. Puffer, chemical conjunctivitis, as this condition is called, may be caused by any of the chemicals used to keep the pool germ free. While the redness won't hurt you, it does indicate an irritation. Your best bet is to avoid it by using goggles. If you swim without them, you may want to use eye drops, such as Murine or Visine, as a temporary soother.

Eye Sunburn

Also known as ultraviolet keratoconjunctivitis, this condition is caused by an overdose of ultraviolet radiation (UV) on the cornea (the clear, protective outer layer of your eye). Water from swimming pools, lakes, or the ocean reflects 85 percent or more UV radiation, so the sun's glare can inflict substantial damage, Dr. Puffer warns.

Like sunburn on your skin, eye sunburn can surface as a delayed reaction, typically 6 to 12 hours after exposure. Your eyes may appear red and irritated and feel gritty and sensitive to light. You may tear a lot and blink uncontrollably. Fortunately, most of this discomfort should disappear within 48 hours. Ophthalmologists usually recommend staying indoors until symptoms disappear.

Your best preventive is a good pair of sunglasses or contacts with adequate UV protection.

Headaches

Sometimes hard play can bring on a headache. Exercise-induced headaches can happen for many different reasons, says Dr. Mellion, who has conducted an extensive review of research on this topic. You may be especially prone if you aren't conditioned enough to play so hard, if you work out too hard at high altitude, if you have uncontrolled diabetes, or if you drink alcohol before or during exercise.

In any case, if your headaches are recurrent or persistent, see a doctor to establish their cause. Sometimes an anti-inflammatory, like aspirin or ibuprofen, can prevent recurrences if you take it before you play.

A cause of headaches in swimmers may sometimes be too much pressure on the forehead and eye sockets, caused by swimming caps or goggles. "Make sure your goggles are well padded," advises Dr. Puffer.

Heat Exhaustion

Have you ever felt clammy, dizzy, and nauseated during the course of a midday jog? You were probably suffering from heat exhaustion. Unlike heatstroke, a life-threatening condition caused when our sweating system shuts down, heat exhaustion occurs when we lose more water through sweat than we take in. It's a drought in the body.

The first thing to do for heat exhaustion is to get to the coolest place around. Keep your feet elevated, loosen your clothing, and drink water. Apply cool, wet cloths, use a fan or move to an air-conditioned room. If the symptoms worsen, get medical help.

To prevent the problem in the first place, drink 1 or 2 cups of water before you even begin your workout, says Dr. Puffer. Stay away from alcoholic beverages. They'll only make you feel warmer, because alcohol calories are burned quickly, raising your metabolic rate and body temperature. "Drink several ounces of cold water every 20 minutes during your game or workout and keep drinking afterward," advises Dr. Puffer. "Drink even more than you're thirsty for."

Finally, when you begin biking, running, or playing tennis in summer heat, cut back on your usual workout until you become acclimated to the change in season.

Intermittent Claudication

This is a cramp in the calves that happens when you walk or run, and is caused by poor circulation due to atherosclerosis (hardening of the arteries) or other artery blockage. It feels like a dull ache and improves dramatically when you're standing still or sitting. If this describes your leg cramps, see your doctor.

Muscle Cramps

Cramps can strike any muscle you overstress, but they usually hit the major muscle groups in your legs: calves, hamstrings, and quadriceps. Rowing your canoe too far, too fast could bring on cramps in your arms, of course, as could swimming too many laps.

"Many muscle cramps are actually a form of heat injury," says Dr. Puffer. "They're one of the first problems we see when the weather gets hot."

What happens is a gradual dehydration. When you sweat, you sweat away fluids and the minerals (or electrolytes) they contain. These minerals are essential for proper muscle function. Failing to drink enough water, your best source of electrolytes, just makes things worse. It's this loss of electrolytes that causes the cramps. The best preventive? "Drink plenty of water—and don't take salt pills. Taking salt pills when you're severely dehydrated can make the concentration of salt in your system too great," says Dr. Mellion. (See "Heat Exhaustion on page 287 for specifics on fluids.)

"Cramps may also attack because a muscle is injured and starts to spasm, and they're especially common in sports where people run a lot," adds Dr. Puffer. "Muscle cramps can even be caused by spasms from overstretching."

The best preventive measure for these spasm cramps is stretching and massage. Dr. Puffer advises a program of stretching both before and after your activity. "Warmed-up muscles are easier to stretch, so get your blood circulating a bit first," he cautions. Make sure to stretch calves, hamstrings, quads, and especially in swimmers, shoulder muscles, adds Dr. Mellion.

The best quick-fix when cramps strike: kneading the muscle.

Muscle Strains

Strains occur when you've stretched your muscles beyond their normal range of movement, usually in the heat of the game when you're throwing caution to the winds. The strained muscle may feel sore or knotted. Rest the muscle and apply ice immediately, says Dr. Puffer. Use aspirin or an aspirin-free painkiller to relieve the pain, but call a doctor if the pain is severe.

Rashes

Those itchy, scaly red marks shaped like a button, a shoe seam, a waistband, or your swim goggles are probably a rash known as contact dermatitis. Heat and sweat make your skin especially vulnerable to allergens, including chemicals that your sweat may leach from your clothing, says dermatologist Rodney Basler, M.D., assistant professor of internal medicine at the University of Nebraska Medical Center. He says that he sees a lot of contact dermatitis caused from rubber in shoes, but rubber or Spandex in the waistbands of swim trunks or jogging shorts can be an irritant, too.

Chemicals in your fabric softener can also cause contact dermatitis, as can the formaldehyde used in fabric sizing. Dr.

Basler recommends washing your new workout clothes at least once before wearing them.

Flexural dermatitis—the rashes you get at points where your body flexes, like elbows and knees—comes from perspiration-trapped allergens. If you have pollen allergies, you may be prone to this rash.

The best prevention is avoiding the allergens in the first place or trying to minimize their impact by reducing the moisture and chafing against your skin, says Dr. Basler. He recommends tucking in your T-shirt to protect your waist. Certain ointments, such as Aquaphor and Eucerin, may help by creating a barrier between your skin and the offending fabric as well as by soothing your skin. Since these ointments are more water soluble than petroleum jelly, they shouldn't get your clothes as greasy. Corticosteroid sprays or ointments, such as Cortaid, may also help.

If your rash becomes severe, your family doctor may prescribe more potent corticosteroids or refer you to a dermatologist for a patch test and further treatment.

Runner's Knee

Dr. Puffer and other experts cite five main causes of the injuries often called "runner's knee." Topping the list are body-alignment problems, most of which can be corrected with shoe orthotics (fitted by an orthopedic or podiatric specialist).

The other four causes are training errors. Changing a training routine too rapidly is the most frequent error. Dr. Puffer advises increasing your mileage gradually, no more than about 10 percent every other week. Speeding up too quickly should also be avoided. Hill work is another major culprit, he notes, especially the run downhill.

"Many problems arise when you overstride as you increase your speed," Dr. Puffer warns. "Shorten your stride and make sure your knees are not completely straight when your feet hit the ground. Flexed knees diffuse the impact of running downhill."

Poor shoes are another source of injury. Dr. Puffer advises buying the best shoes you can afford if you're going to take up running regularly. You can check your shoes for wear by setting them on a countertop so you can view them at eye level.

Finally, Dr. Puffer advises that you avoid running on hard surfaces.

If your knees begin to hurt, Dr. Puffer advises seeing a doctor to find out exactly what's causing it. The best interim treatment is RICE, an acronym for rest (stop all activity); ice (wrap it in a towel and apply to the injured area for 20 minutes to reduce swelling; repeat as needed); compression (wrap with an Ace bandage); and elevation (raise the limb to drain it of excess fluid). Your doctor may recommend quadriceps-strengthening exercises to protect your knees from further injury.

Saddle Sores

Saddles, whether on a bike or a horse, can chafe the novice or infrequent rider, causing uncomfortable lesions where you grip the horse or rub against the bike seat. The cyclist's best protection is a well-padded seat, says Dr. Puffer, and both horseback riders and cyclists can benefit by wearing suitable clothing. Novice or infrequent horseback riders should not depend on jeans for extended riding on an English saddle, for example. If you can't spring for jodhpurs, at least wear pants with lightweight seams. The heavy French seams in most jeans can rub your legs the wrong way. Likewise, cyclists who plan to log a lot of distance in the saddle are best off buying cycling shorts, which are designed to be worn without chafing underwear.

Shoulder Tendinitis

If you overdo any sport where you swing your arms over-head, you can cause tears and inflammation in the muscles and tendons that support and hold together your shoulder's ball-and-socket joint. This is known as shoulder, or rotator-cuff, tendinitis.

The best preventive is cutting back on moves that contribute little to your fitness level but increase your risk of injury. Cut back on extra laps, swings, or serves by varying your activities, mixing tennis with jogging or walking, for example, or other activities that don't use overhead arm motions. Baseball pitchers should limit practice sessions, trade off games with another pitcher, and warm up carefully before every game.

Rest is the best cure for tendinitis. You may also want to apply an ice pack for about 15 to 20 minutes after you first experience pain. If pain persists beyond the next two days or so, your doctor may prescribe an anti-inflammatory drug.

Side Stitches

"Side stitches are probably spasms in the diaphragm," Dr. Puffer explains. "They are more common in poorly conditioned people than well-conditioned athletes, and they tend to strike when you're breathing too fast." The best preventive *and* remedy is to slow your pace, taking slow, even breaths.

Sprains

Sprains happen when you've stretched or torn a ligament, usually by overextending or twisting a joint. The injured area could be painful, swollen, tender to the touch, or discolored. Dr. Puffer advises that you keep the joint still. If the injury is to an ankle or knee, remove the shoe and apply RICE as for "Runner's Knee" on page 290. If your wrist has been sprained, bandage and elevate it; if an elbow or shoulder, put it in a sling. "Don't assume any injury is a simple sprain," says Dr. Puffer. "Go see a doctor for a proper diagnosis."

Swimmer's Ear

The throbbing pain in the ear that some swimmers get often comes from too much time under water. When your ear canal has been soaking in water too long, Dr. Puffer explains, it begins to lose its protective wax coating, making it vulnerable to infection. To help deter infection, try a simple solution of 1 part alcohol to 3 parts hydrogen peroxide, he says. A drop in each ear before you swim should disinfect the ear canal and help the water evaporate quickly. Once you've become infected, see a doctor for treatment instead of waiting it out.

Tennis Elbow

If the ping of ball against racket is accompanied by a pang in the elbow, you may have tennis elbow. The pain occurs on the inside surface of the elbow and is caused by serving too hard over too long a period. As with back injuries, the keys to prevention are correct form, properly fitted equipment, and flexibility and strengthening exercises.

Proper form is crucial. A lesson or two at the beginning of the season should help correct any unhealthy habits. The most common error is failing to keep your eye on the ball, causing you to hit weakly or off-center, which is especially jarring to your elbow. Your pro may suggest a Jimmy Connors-style two-handed backhand to help prevent injury.

Dr. Puffer says that light to light-medium weight wood or graphite rackets with the weight centered more toward the handle than the head absorb impact best. Head-heavy rackets strain the underdeveloped wrist and forearm. Flexible rackets absorb shock. Oversized rackets have larger sweet spots so you have a better chance to hit the ball with minimum resistance. String the racket at 50- to 54-pound tension, and use gut instead of nylon. Grip size is key. Your pro shop can help determine your proper grip size.

Dr. Puffer recommends using weights to strengthen your wrist, elbow, forearm, and shoulder.

Tennis Toe

Tennis toe looks like a bruise or a black spot under the toenail of your big toe. It's usually caused by toenails that are too long, by poorly fitted shoes, or by sudden stops and turns that force your toenail into the front of your (properly fitted) shoe. The impact can cause a loosened nail and a hemorrhage.

A doctor can relieve the pressure of the trapped fluids by burning through the nail with an instrument called the Geiger cautery. Rest and warm water soaks help chronic cases. Preventive measures: Regularly trim your toenails straight across, almost to the quick, and wear shoes that fit well.

Chase Away the Chills

What cold problem is more common than the common cold? The answer is in your hands—and your feet. Everyone is bothered to some degree by cold hands and feet, but in most cases this cold condition is easier to remedy than sniffles and sneezes.

Most commonly, frigid fingers and toes result from a he-moglobin detour. When your core body temperature drops, your nervous system makes the tiny blood vessels around your hands and feet constrict. That redirects warming blood to a more important place, the internal organs.

Help for cold digits ranges from high-tech to low. Keep in mind, too, that certain medications can cool your body temper-ature. Consult your physician or pharmacist if you suspect a problem. Beyond that, there are a number of simple remedies anyone can benefit from. Here are some of the best chill-chasers.

Iron It Out

All houses aren't insulated the same; neither are people. Some are more susceptible to cold hands and feet because their core body temperature is set lower or is more easily lowered than others. For instance, a woman's core body temperature is set 3 to 4 degrees lower than a man's, so women are more likely to get cold hands and feet.

Another reason that women might be naturally colder than men (and thus have colder hands and feet) is lack of iron. Most women between the ages of 11 and 50 fail to consume the recommended 18 milligrams of iron a day, and two researchers recently linked iron deficiency with lower core body tempera-ture. (Iron plays an important role in forming hemoglobin, which helps blood carry oxygen to the tissues.)

At Pennsylvania State University, John Beard, Ph.D., created an experiment that looked like a sorority prank—he had anemic and nonanemic women sit in lawn chairs, sub-merged to the neck in 82°F water. But the results were no joke: He found that the anemic women generated 13 percent less body heat than the nonanemic women.

Meanwhile, at the USDA Human Nutrition Research Center in Grand Forks, North Dakota, the effects of dietary iron were measured in six healthy women who entered a 64°F chamber. When the women took only a third of the recom-mended amount of iron for 80 days, they lost 29 percent more body heat than when they were on an iron-replete diet for 114 days. They also reported more trouble sleeping when in the iron-reduced state, according to Henry Lukaski, Ph.D., who headed the study.

Both researchers believe that iron deficiency somehow alters thyroid metabolism, which regulates body heat. The meaning of all this hasn't been totally ironed out yet. But for now, Dr. Lukaski recommends eating iron-rich foods like fish, poultry, lean red meat, lentils, and green leafy vegetables. And wash them down with orange juice: Vitamin C increases the body's ability to absorb iron.

Wind Up When the Wind's Up

You can actually force your hands to warm up through a simple exercise that Donald McIntyre, M.D., a dermatologist in Rutland, Vermont, devised. Pretend you're a souped-up softball pitcher: Swing your arm downward behind your body and then upward in front of you at about 80 twirls per minute (this isn't as fast as it sounds; give it a try).

The windmill effect, which Dr. McIntyre modeled after a skiers' warm-up exercise, forces blood to the fingers through both gravitational and centrifugal force. This warm-up works well for chilled hands and feet no matter what the cause is— even if it's Raynaud's syndrome, a mysterious hand-chilling phenomenon. And it works fast: A 40-year-old man was able to reverse a Raynaud's attack after 90 seconds of twirling his arms.

Dress Smart

To keep warm you have to dress warmly. Common sense, yes, but many people will slap on gloves and footwear without taking equal precautions to maintain their core temperature, which is really more important. Another common mistake: dressing too warmly, with nonbreathable materials.

The fact is, perspiration is an even bigger cause of cold hands and feet than temperature. Sweat is the body's natural air conditioner, and your body's air conditioner can operate even in cold weather if you're not careful. The hands and feet are especially susceptible because the palms and heels (along with the armpits) have the largest number of sweat glands in the body. That's why the heavy woolen socks and fleece-lined boots you bought to keep your feet warm may instead make them sweaty and chilly.

If you're stepping out into the cold, the best warming measure you can take is to dress in layers. This helps trap heat and allows you to peel off clothes as the temperature changes. Your inner layer should consist of one of the new synthetic fabrics, like polypropylene, that wicks perspiration away from your skin. Silk or wool blends are acceptable as well. The next layer should insulate you by trapping your body heat. A wool shirt or sweater is one of your best options. Your outermost layer should protect you against the elements and allow perspiration to evaporate, so choose a breathable, waterproof jacket or windbreaker.

Wear socks that wick moisture away from your feet and insulate them. All-cotton socks can soak up your perspiration and chill your feet. Those made of Orlon and cotton are a better option.

Choose your footwear carefully, too. Gore-Tex shoes and boots are the best choice for keeping your feet warm and dry.

None of your garments should pinch. Tight-fitting clothes, whether they are nylons, garter belts, jeans, or shoes, can cut off circulation and eliminate insulating air pockets.

The single best piece of clothing you can wear to warm your hands and feet is a hat. Your head is the greatest site of body heat loss. The blood vessels in your head are controlled by cardiac output and won't constrict like those in your hands and feet. In fact, John Abruzzo, M.D., director of rheumatology at Thomas Jefferson University in Philadelphia, says that if you want to keep your hands and feet warm, it's as important to wear a hat as it is to wear gloves and socks.

Finally, mittens are preferable to gloves because they trap the heat from your whole hands.

Dry Up

Clothes aren't the only way to keep dry. "Absorbent foot powders are excellent for helping keep feet dry," says Marc A. Brenner, D.P.M., past president of the American Society of

Podiatric Dermatology. But he cautions people with severe cold-feet problems caused by diabetes and peripheral vascular disease to use a shaker can rather than an aerosol spray, since the mist from the spray can actually freeze their feet.

Douse It

Smokers set themselves up for cold hands and feet whenever they light up. Cigarette smoke cools you two ways: It helps form plaque in your arteries and, more immediately, even one puff of nicotine causes vasospasms that narrow the small blood vessels. These effects can be especially hard on people with Raynaud's. "Raynaud's patients are sensitive even to other people's smoke," says Frederick A. Reichle, M.D., chief of vascular surgery at Presbyterian-University of Pennsylvania Medical Center.

Chill Out to Warm Up

Staying cool and calm may actually help some people stay warm. Reason: Stress creates the same reaction in the body as cold. It's the fight-or-flight phenomenon—blood is pulled from the hands and feet to the brain and internal organs to enable you to think and react more quickly.

Calming techniques abound. Some, like progressive relaxation—in which you systematically tense, then relax the muscles from your forehead to your hands and toes—can be practiced any time, any place.

Warm Up with a Hot Meal

The very act of eating causes a rise in core body temperature. This is called thermogenesis. So eat something before you go out, to stoke your body's furnace. And eat something hot to give the stoking a boost. A bowl of hot oatmeal before your morning walk, a soup break or hot lunch will help keep your hands and feet toasty even in inclement weather.

Drink Up

Dehydration can aggravate chills and frostbite by reducing your blood volume. So ward off the big chill by drinking plenty of fluids such as hot cider, herbal teas, or broth. Avoid caffeine-containing beverages, however, since caffeine constricts blood vessels. And don't be misled by the lure of a hot toddy, either. A touch of alcohol will temporarily warm up your hands and feet, but the drug's detrimental effects outweigh its benefits as a hand and foot warmer.

Alcohol increases blood flow to the skin (this is why heavy drinkers like the late W. C. Fields are noted for their red noses), giving you the immediate perception of warmth. But that heat is soon lost to the air, reducing your core body temperature so the alcohol is actually making you colder. The danger comes from drinking an immodest amount and being subjected to unexpected cold for an extended period, which can lead to severe problems, like frostbite. Says Dr. Abruzzo, "The model of the St. Bernard dog with a flask of brandy around his neck is an unfortunate one."

Check for Raynaud's

If your fingertips turn white, blue, and red, you may be suffering from Raynaud's syndrome. In Raynaud's, the blood vessels to the extremities can constrict even before the core body temperature begins to fall. (In severe cases, simply opening a refrigerator door can set off an attack.) Raynaud's also can be triggered by vibrations—such as operating a sledgehammer or typing.

No one knows how common Raynaud's is because many people don't consider the condition serious enough to bring it to their doctor's attention. Indeed, Raynaud's is often more of a bother than a serious medical problem. But the condition is treatable. See your doctor if your fingers are painful or change colors.

The U.S. Army recently perfected a simple technique that allows Raynaud's sufferers to train their bodies to overcome chills. The technique, which Army researchers in Alaska began fiddling with ten years ago, is based on the same principle Pavlov used in training dogs to salivate at the sound of a bell.

The canines began licking their chops because they learned to associate the bell with chow time; in the Army exercise, people learned to condition their hands to warm up when the weather turned cold. Here's how it works: Starting at room temperature, place your hands in a container of warm water. Then go into a freezing room and again dip your hands in warm water, for 10 minutes. The cold environment would normally make your peripheral blood vessels constrict; instead, the sensation of the warm water makes them open. Repeatedly training the blood vessels to open despite the cold eventually enables you to counter the constriction reflex even without the warm water.

In the Army experiments, this procedure was repeated every other day for three to six times on 150 test subjects. After 54 treatments, the subjects' results were impressive: Their hands were 7 degrees warmer in the cold than before.

Taking a warm-water dip is far easier than other treatments for severe Raynaud's, such as drug therapy. "People are training on the rooftops in New York City, in freezer lockers, in grocery stores, and in hospitals and hotels," says Murray Hamlet, director of the Army's cold-research program.

Cater to Your Stomach's Quirks

Good digestion isn't as simple as chewing an after-dinner mint. If it were, diverticular disease, irritable bowel syndrome, heartburn, hemorrhoids, gas, and flatulence—some of the most common digestive problems—would never arise.

But arise they do. And that after-dinner mint may be a contributing factor. So, instead of mints, here's a healthy serving of all the best current advice to keep your digestion on track. Bon appetit.

The Ins and Outs of Gas

Doctors call it aerophagia. The name sounds like a Soviet airline. It means air swallowing—the cause, says experts, of most belching. Gulp. We all do it, especially when stressed. Swallow enough and we swell up and—ah, relief!—belch.

Belching, however, begets belching. A belch is often followed by more air swallowing and another belch. But even chronic air swallowers can break the habit. For a businessman who swallowed air and bloated painfully at important meetings, Marvin Schuster, M.D., a professor at Johns Hopkins University School of Medicine in Baltimore, prescribed a pencil. "Clamping your teeth around a pencil—or a cork or your finger—keeps your mouth open and makes swallowing difficult," he says.

Some swallowed air finds its way into the intestines. That's where the other gas—flatus—comes in. And, eventually, comes out.

Most flatus is caused by colonic bacteria, which ferment undigested food and create gas as a by-product. The odor comes from hydrogen sulfide (of rotten-egg fame), fatty acids, and other compounds—rather potent substances detectable by smell in 1 part per 100 million.

Because bacteria vary among people, so do flatus-inspiring foods. Almost everybody gets flatus from beans. They contain the starches raffinose and stachyose, which bacteria ferment vigorously. (Beans can be degassed, though. See "Prepping Beans for Digestion.")

One study found onions, celery, carrots, raisins, bananas, apricots, prune juice, bagels, pretzels, wheat germ, and brussels sprouts highly flatugenic. High-fiber foods can also be a problem, particularly if you suddenly increase them in your diet.

"Start with a small dose of fiber so the bowel gets used to it," says Michael Mogadam, M.D., of Georgetown University in Washington D.C. "That lessens the increase in flatus." Anyway, most people's flatus production returns to normal within a few weeks of adding fiber.

Crescendos of 141 passages per day—including 70 in 4 hours—have been documented in severe cases of flatulence. Average in seven 28-year-old men tested by Michael D. Levitt, M.D., of Minneapolis Veterans Administration Hospital, was 14, plus or minus 5, per day.

Severe flatulence—the 141-a-day case, for instance—is sometimes linked to lactose intolerance. Lactose-intolerant people lack the enzyme lactase, needed to digest the milk sugar, or lactose. It arrives in their colons undigested and ripe for fermentation.

PREPPING BEANS FOR DIGESTION

Beans have a bad reputation for producing gas. The problem is they contain certain water-soluble starches that the body cannot break down during digestion. But the key here is "water-soluble." By repeatedly soaking the beans in water (and discarding the runoff), much of the problem can be eliminated. Here's how.

1. Start with a pound (2 cups) of dried beans. Discard any that are broken or discolored. Rinse until the water runs clear.

2. Place the beans in a large soup pot with 6 cups of cold water. Boil for 2 minutes.

3. Drain the water and replace it with fresh. Let stand overnight or for at least 6 hours.

4. Drain well. Add fresh water. Bring to a boil, then simmer, loosely covered, until the legumes are tender (start checking lentils after 30 minutes; others will take up to 2 hours).

To save time, you can prepare the beans ahead of time and store for later use. Beans prepared as above can keep for a week in the refrigerator or 6 months in the freezer. (Don't freeze lentils, however; they turn mushy.)

To test for intolerance, avoid all dairy products, including dry milk solids and whey, for two weeks. If flatus decreases, intolerance is the problem. The solution? Less lactose.

If other steps don't curb excessive flatulence, doctors may prescribe simethicone, said to break up bubbles and make them easier to expel. Activated charcoal seems to be a better choice. It soaks up gas until excreted in stool. A double-blind, placebo-controlled study of nine adults found simethicone had little effect. But charcoal significantly reduced flatus production and abdominal symptoms. (Keep in mind, however, that charcoal can soak up medicine, too, blocking its effectiveness. If you take medication, check with a doctor before trying charcoal.)

In the end, flatus is a social problem, not a medical one. Don't worry about flatus if it doesn't bother you, recommends

B. R. Cohen, M.D., of Mount Sinai Medical Center in New York City.

Spelling Relief—With and without Antacids

It may feel like a lead weight on your sternum. Or a too-tight bra. More often, though, it simply burns inside the chest. Heart attack? No, heartburn—one of the most common reasons people see gastroenterologists. Blame heartburn on the lower esophageal sphincter: the smooth, cylinder-shaped muscle at the junction of the esophagus and stomach. As a one-way valve, it opens to drop in food and closes to keep acid from coming back. It's supposed to, anyway.

But when the valve opens at the wrong time or doesn't close completely, bile from the small intestine and pepsin and gastric acid from the stomach squirt into the acid-sensitive esophagus.

Changing eating habits is the best way to prevent heartburn, says Joel Richter, M.D., of Wake Forest University in Winston-Salem, North Carolina. Start with smaller meals. They leave the stomach quickly, producing less acid than large meals.

Cut down on dietary fats, too. They prompt the release of hormones that present a double threat. First, they decrease stomach emptying and increase acid. Second, the hormones open the lower esophageal sphincter. After-dinner chocolates, peppermints, and liqueurs pack the same double whammy.

Nonalcoholic drinks, too, cause heartburn in some people. Coffee and tea stimulate acid output. Citrus and tomato juices can irritate the esophagus.

As if that's not enough, people react individually to foods. Onions and cabbage give some of us heartburn (not to mention flatulence), but don't bother others. Keeping track of diet and symptoms with a diary can uncover problem foods. Avoiding them reduces heartburn.

To prevent late-night heartburn, don't sleep with a full stomach. Acid peaks in the 2 hours after each meal. So if possible, go to bed on an empty stomach and sleep with the head of your bed raised 6 inches. Gravity helps keep stomach acid down.

Antacids, of course, can take the sting out of heartburn. Liquids, and to a lesser extent, pills neutralize stomach acid, so it stops irritating the esophagus.

If heartburn persists in spite of antacids and changed eating habits, see a physician. A doctor can prescribe drugs like cimetidine (Tagamet) or ranitidine (Zantac), which lower the stomach's acid production.

Another digestive problem, irritable bowel syndrome (IBS) is collection of unpleasant symptoms: constipation, diarrhea, flatulence, painful bloating, gas, nausea. Although it accounts for half their referrals—women with the syndrome outnumber men three to one—gastroenterologists don't know what causes IBS. They do know that stress seems to trigger symptoms.

There are two major types of IBS. In one, patients have urgent diarrhea first thing in the morning or during or after meals. In the other, they experience painful constipation, diarrhea, or alternating bouts of each. Fatigue, depression, and anxiety often accompany the physical symptoms.

But IBS isn't all in the mind. It's also in the gut. Bowel muscles may contract up to nine times a minute instead of the normal three, stretching the intestinal wall. That's the source of the pain.

Although IBS has no known cure, most people can learn to manage the symptoms. The best way, says Dr. Richter, is by reducing stress. Vigorous, regular exercise—for those who are able—helps do just that. It releases endorphins, opiate-like brain chemicals that lessen anxiety. Some types of exercise—curl-ups, for instance—also help the bowel. "When you bend back and forth, the colon bends, too," says Dr. Mogadam. "That helps provoke peristalsis [normal intestinal contractions] and relieves the spasms in the bowel. That's very helpful for constipated people."

Diet is the other key to controlling IBS. As with heartburn, a diet diary can uncover irritating foods. Reduce fatty foods, since they can stimulate excessive muscle contractions. Protein, on the other hand, may decrease them.

A high-fiber diet can help, too. But watch out for beans and other flatugenics.

Although IBS can be painful and uncomfortable, it isn't life-threatening. If pain, diarrhea, or constipation become unmanageable, though, see a doctor.

Some doctors think there's a link between long-term IBS and the development of diverticula, small outpouchings in the colon ranging from the size of a piece of confetti to a that of a quarter. Between 30 and 40 percent of people over age 50 have them.

Diverticula aren't the problem. Trouble starts when they become infected and inflamed, a condition called diverticulitis. High pressure in the colon (caused by straining) can create a tiny hole in a diverticulum, where bacteria or feces lodge. That means infection, inflammation, and pain. In extreme cases, the condition can become life-threatening.

The best thing to keep diverticula from starting or getting worse is a high-fiber diet, doctors say. It widens the colon a bit, keeping pressure low. Increase fiber (bran cereal and whole wheat bread are recommended) gradually, though. Too much too soon can mean bloating and flatulence.

A Fit Ending

Nobody sings the praises of anal or rectal blood vessels. But maybe somebody should. They act like inflatable cushions, forming a tight seal that prevents stool from leaking from the rectum. Sometimes, though, the cushions overinflate, becoming hemorrhoids.

What makes them act up? Gravity, which pulls blood downward.

An ounce of prevention is worth a pound of Preparation H. Moderate exercise, such as walking, keeps blood moving and the blood vessels from overinflating. William Stern, M.D., of George Washington University, also recommends fiber. It stops constipation and hemorrhoids before they start.

Once hemorrhoids develop, itching and pain can be minimized. When there's discomfort without bleeding, over-the-counter suppositories or ointments often do the trick. Though they don't cure hemorrhoids, they lubricate the rectum and anus, making hard stools pass easier. "Natural" bulk-forming laxatives like those made with psyllium (Metamucil, for instance) reduce constipation and the abrasion and straining it causes.

Warm baths help shrink swollen tissue. Dr. Stern recommends patients take two baths daily and apply cream after each.

For bleeding, though, a visit to the doctor is imperative. Blood on the stool or toilet paper could be related to other serious problems, such as polyps or even colon cancer.

See a doctor, too, if hemorrhoids interfere with daily activity. Doctors can repair them in the office with infrared, ultroid (electric-current) or cryosurgery (freezing)—even rubber bands. All these restrict blood flow, destroying the hemorrhoid.

Filling Out without Fattening Up

By George L. Blackburn, M.D., Ph.D.

Gaining weight: It's a challenge many of us would love to face. Yet, gaining weight can involve as much effort as losing, especially if you are concerned about your health.

After all, gaining 10 pounds won't do much for your health or your looks if those pounds are added as fat. What you should aim for is gaining muscle mass. And for that, it takes the right kind of diet and exercise.

Who Stands to Gain?

First, make sure that you really could benefit from gaining weight—not everyone who thinks he or she needs to gain really does. If you feel energetic all day long, then sleep well and wake up feeling great, if you have enough upper-body strength to tote suitcases and children or grandchildren, then your light weight is probably not a problem. You're just naturally thin.

If, however, you became thin because of an eating disorder or illness, if you do feel weak and lack energy, or if you'd like to try to build yourself up for strength, endurance, and looks, weight gain is for you.

Just be sure to consult a health professional for guidance.

Most people think that the key to weight gain is to eat a lot more than they usually do. But that's a myth. You actually need only about 100 to 200 extra calories each day to build and sustain the muscle tissue that you will develop in your exercise program.

And while you might feel that this is the perfect opportunity to pig out on milk shakes and hot-fudge sundaes, don't do it. Quality is as important as quantity in a weight-gain diet. Excess fat in the diet causes excess fat on your body and in the long run can lead to serious health problems, such as heart disease.

The extra calories should come from healthy, low-fat foods—interestingly, the same foods you should eat on a weight-loss diet: grain products such as breads, pasta and cereals, low-fat dairy products such as skim milk, yogurt and cottage cheese, and protein foods such as chicken (without the skin), fish, and lean meat.

Do not be tempted by the protein supplements that are heavily marketed to professional body builders, however. They deliver excess protein, which has the potential to harm your kidneys.

If you're not sure how to make these changes, consult a registered dietitian knowledgeable about body building. He or she can help you find simple ways to adjust your diet.

Build Up Your Body

Remember, too: Diet is only half the battle. To build muscle—not just get fat—you've got to exercise, too. And not just any kind will do. While aerobic exercise is excellent for cardiovascular conditioning, it alone can't produce the kind of muscle development that shows up in added pounds on the scale. For that, you need circuit training—a combination of calisthenics (such as push-ups), weight training, stretching, and aerobic exercise.

Consult a physician in a sports-medicine practice or seek out a certified exercise instructor to design the program that's right for you.

And be prepared to give your muscle-building program plenty of time. You'll have to work at it consistently for 6 to 12 months to see a big difference. But it will be worth the effort because the benefits of body building go beyond curing skinniness, especially for mature women. Many women lack upper-body strength, which becomes more of a problem as they get older. Strong and flexible muscles can help you prevent a fall or catch yourself if you do fall. And regular exercise may help deter osteoporosis. Another benefit: A strong back and chest improves your breathing.

The Setpoint Dilemma

Not everyone who wants to gain weight can. Each of us has a "setpoint," determined by individual genetics, physiology, and metabolism of working muscles. If your setpoint wants you thin, you may find that even a properly implemented diet and exercise program won't beef you up to your expectations. If that's the case, accept it, and enjoy the envy of friends who ask you, "How do you stay so slender?"

The Fine Art of Face Washing

Why do so many of us spend so much time selecting and using just the right moisturizer or makeup, yet spend only 2 minutes washing our face with the same product we use on our hands? Let's put first things first. Let's get the most out of those moisturizers and makeup by starting with a proper cleansing program customized to our skin's needs.

Choosing a Cleanser

According to New York City dermatologist Ronald Sherman, M.D., two things that any cleanser must do are clean thoroughly and clean gently.

If you have sensitive or dry skin, look for a gentle nonsoap cleanser or a soap substitute specifically for the face. Shun the alkaline body or deodorant soaps. They generally contain fatty acids neutralized with lye or harsh detergents with ingredients that can strip your complexion of essential natural oils, or both.

Don't get the idea, though, that *detergent* is necessarily a dirty word. "A 'detergent' soap is simply a synthetic soap," says Dr. Sherman. "It can be harsh or gentle, depending on which chemical ingredient is added. The varying formulas allow manufacturers to make soaps to fill the needs of each skin type. Almost all the soaps you can think of, including the mildest like Dove, are detergents."

"If your skin is normal, the goal of cleansing is to keep it that way," says Joseph Melnik, director of research and development for Erno Laszlo skin-care products. "All you need is a mild soap that rinses off easily." Like people with dry or sensitive skin, you should avoid harsh deodorant soaps.

If you have oily skin, you need a cleansing routine that leaves a balanced complexion neither too dry nor too oily. Try one of the transparent soaps that contain glycerin and alcohol.

"It's important to keep in mind that within each general skin type there are degrees of dry, normal, and oily, and these can change with the seasons," adds Dr. Sherman. "Someone who has dry skin will be drier in the winter, and someone who has an oily complexion will have to deal with more oil in the summer. The bottom line here is that you have to monitor your own skin and be ready to alter your skin-care program."

The Good Wash

How you cleanse your face can be as important as what you use. First, secure your hair completely off your face. Terry-cloth headbands work great (use athletic sweatbands or strips of towel).

Then fill the basin with warm water and wet your face with clean hands. "We recommend using your hands because washcloths generally aren't really clean, plus they tend to be more abrasive," says Melnik. With your hands, work the cleanser up into a good lather and gently massage it into your face and throat.

"Don't rub too hard," says Dr. Sherman. "Some people seem to be trying to erase their face, as if by scrubbing hard enough they can take off their own face and find Elizabeth

Taylor." Roughing up your skin just irritates it. No scrubbing allowed.

If you can't get used to washing with your hands alone, baby your face with the flannel washcloths designed for infants. "For optimum cleanliness, use a new flannel each day," says Melnik.

Rinsing Right

Do you place your soapy washcloth under running water for a few seconds, then rinse your face with it? Most people do. But this perfunctory rinse leaves cleanser and dirt on your facecloth and on your face. And this residue can dry your complexion, leaving it feeling taut and looking dull. If you've got dry skin and are using a cleansing cream, half-hearted rinsing will leave behind a mixture of cream and dirt that may cause blemishes.

"The cleanser breaks up the grime, oil, and makeup that are on your face and prepares them to be removed, but you must rinse off every trace of this cleanser/dirt mixture," says Melnik. "Cleansing products tend to be surface active, which means if they're left on, they can penetrate the skin, carrying oil and grime with them."

Melnik recommends rinsing with your bare hands at least 25 times in a sink of warm water, and another 10 times with running water. You should feel your skin become completely free of any soap residue. Don't miss the hairline area and around the jawline.

It may take a few tries before you can do this without splashing water all over the bathroom and yourself. It may help to put your face as close to the water as possible instead of trying to bring the water up to your face.

Pat or blot dry. "Men tend to blot their skin, while women tend to rub theirs, especially around the eyes," says Dr. Sherman. "But this rubbing around the eyes and on the eyelid can cause a lot of irritation there."

Toning Up

The next step is applying a toner. All toners, also called fresheners or astringents, depending on which complexion they're formulated for, are used to help remove the last traces of cleanser, exfoliate (remove dead skin cells), and soothe. The only difference between astringents and fresheners is that astringents contain more alcohol and thus are more drying than fresheners.

Saturate a cotton ball with your toner and sweep it lightly over your face, avoiding the eye area. This is also a good test of how well you're cleansing. If there's more than just a trace of dirt or oil on the cotton, rethink the first three steps of your cleansing program. Either your cleanser isn't doing its job, you're not hitting all areas of your face evenly, or you're not rinsing thoroughly enough. Diagnose your problem and correct it.

Don't depend on the toning step of your program to "mop up" after your cleanser. Toners, if overused, can strip even oily skin of necessary natural oil.

Index

A

Abdominal muscles, 179
Acquired immune deficiency
  syndrome. *See* AIDS
Aerobics, 9, 179
Aerophagia, 299–302
Age, sleep and, 206
Aging
  abdominal muscles and, 179
  aerobic capacity and, 179
  alcohol consumption and, 176
  calories and, 176
  coffee drinking and, 174–75
  exercise and, 179, 181
  flexibility and, 177, 179
  metabolic rate and, 181
  metabolic slowdown and, 176
  middle-age spread and, 179
  muscle conditioning and, 177
  nutrition and, 173–74
  tea drinking and, 174–75
  tendon conditioning and, 177
  weight loss and, 176–77
AIDS
  acquiring
    known ways of, 201
    risks for, 202
  acupuncture and, 199
  Belle Glade scare, 200
  breath and, 197
  coughing and, 198
  direct inoculation and, 201
  donating blood and, 199
  ear piercing and, 199
  eating in restaurants and, 199
  fear of, 197
  French kissing and, 199
  gamma-globulin injection and,
    200
  hepatitis-B vaccine and, 200
  hot tubs and, 198–99
  household members and, 201
  hugging and, 198
  kissing and, 199
  mosquitoes and, 200
  pets and, 200
  protection against, 197
  receiving blood infected with,
    199
  saliva and, 198
  sex and, 202–3
  shaking hands and, 198
  sneezing and, 198
  swimming pools and, 198–99
  tattooing and, 199
  toilet seats and, 198
  unsterilized needles and, 199
Air conditioners, indoor air pollution
  and, 190–93
Air pollution, indoor
  air conditioners and, 190–93
  allergens and, 196–97
  ductwork and, 192–93
  in energy efficient homes,
    196–97
  formaldehyde and, 195–96
  heating and, 193–95
  radon, 196
Alcoholic beverages
  breast cancer and, 12
  calories in, 176
  high-density lipoprotein and, 221
  hypertension and, 79, 167
Aldalactone, magnesium and, 146
Allergies, 267–69
ALS. *See* Amyotrophic lateral
  sclerosis
Amblyopia, 225
Amiloride, magnesium and, 146
Amino acids, 149–53
Amyotrophic lateral sclerosis (ALS),
  149–50
Ancrod, blood clots and, 1
Anemia, 122
Anger, hypertension and, 171
Antacids for heartburn, 302–3
Antibiotics, frogs and, 161
Anticancer drugs, 160–61
Anticancer foods, 54–61. *See also*
  specific foods
Antihistamines, rub-on, 267–68
Antioxidants, 135–36
Anxiety, insomnia and, 207
Applesauce Muffins, 118–19
Apricots, 56
Arginine, muscles and, 150–52
Arrhythmias, magnesium and,
  143–44

Artemisia annua, malaria and, 161
Arthritis. *See also* Osteoarthritis
  description of, 69–70
  fish oil and, 2, 71–72
  primrose oil and, 2
  walking and, 233–35
Aspirin in TMJ disorders, 273
Asthma, 9, 17
Autism, vitamin B$_6$ and, 155–56

B
Backache, 264–65
  cycling and, 283–84
  exercises for, 265–67
  flexibility and, 265
  golf and, 284
  swimming and, 283–84
  tennis and, 284
Bananas, vitamin B$_6$ in, 158
Beans
  as anticancer food, 58–59
  cholesterol and, 62–63
  iron in, 124–25
  preparation of, to decrease gas,
    301
  recipes for, 68–69
Belching, 299–300
Beta-carotene, cancer and, 55,
  127–29
Bikini bottom, 284
Birth control. *See* Contraception
Birth defects, 18
Blisters, 285
Blood clots, snake venom and, 1
Blood pressure. *See also*
  Hypertension
  garlic and, 74
  measurement of, regular, 170
  medication for, 172
  reduction of
    family members and, 172
    recipes for, 80, 82, 83,
      84, 85
    strategies for, 165–73
  walking and, 229–30
Blood transfusion, 199, 201
Body conditioning, middle age and,
  177, 179
Bone(s), 133
  boron and, 134–35
  density of, walking and, 4
  exercise and, 165
Bone marrow cancer, 260–61
Boredom, middle age and, 187
Boron, effect of, on bones, 134–35
Bran cereal, 56

Brazil nuts, 56
Bread, whole wheat, 61
Breakfast
  vitamin B$_6$ in, 158
  weight loss and, 107–8
Breast cancer, 12, 87–91
Broccoli, 57
Brown rice, 57
Brussels sprouts, 57
Bruxism, 7
Butternut squash, 57

C
Cabbage, 54, 57
Cactus, diabetes and, 161
Caffeine, TMJ disorders and, 274
Calcium
  cancer and, 56, 132
    current research on, 132–33
  excess protein and, 164
  getting enough, 162–63
  hypertension and, 79
  inhibition of iron absorption by,
    124
  oxylate and absorption of, 164
  phosphate and, 163–64
  soft drinks and, 163–64
Calluses, 286
Calmness, hypertension and, 172
Calories
  in foods, 176
  weight loss and, 100–101
Camphor, 260–61
Cancer. *See also specific types;*
Anticancer foods.
  beta-carotene and, 55, 127–29
  cabbage family and, 54
  calcium and, 56, 132–33
  cruciferous vegetables and, 54
  fiber and, 55
  low-fat diet and, 55
  magnesium and, 146
  mutant fungi and, 160–61
  omega-3 fats and, 52
  research, 260–63
  risk for, 89
  selenium and, 55–56, 131
  vegetables and, 54
  vitamin A and, 55, 127–29
  vitamin C and, 54–55, 129–30
  vitamin E and, 55, 130
Canola oil, 58
Cantaloupe, 57
Carbon monoxide, 193
Cardiovascular disease, 139–40
Cardiovascular system, 181

Carpal tunnel syndrome (CTS), 156–57
Carrots, 57
Cataracts, 136–37
Cauliflower, 57
Cereal, bran, 56
Chard, 57
Chicken breast, 58
Chicken/Garbanzo Sandwich, 68–69
Chili Con Carne, 69
Chills, 293–95, 297–98
Chlorothiazide, magnesium and, 146
Cholesterol
    coffee and, 174
    fats and, 217–18
    in foods, 217
    hardening of the arteries and, 221
    high-density lipoprotein, 20, 221, 229–30
    high-mono diet and, 14
    low-density lipoprotein, 38
    lowering high levels of
        diet strategies for, 64–66
        drugs for, 221–22
        recipes for, 67–69
    magnesium and, 144–45
    omega-3 fats and, 218
    questions and answers on, 216–22
    soluble fiber and, 62–63
    tea and, 174
    test for, 220–21
    in vegetable oils, 217
Cholestyramine, 222
Cigarette smoking
    chills and, 297
    hypertension and, 172
    indoor air pollution and, 195
    nonsmokers and, 210–16
    vitamin E and, 141–42
Circulatory system, garlic and, 74
Claudication, intermittent, 288
Coffee, 125, 174–75
Cold(s)
    garlic and, 74–75
    TMJ disorders and, 274–75
Colestid, 222
Colestipol, 222
Collard greens, 58
Colon cancer, reduced risk of, 19
Communication, walking and, 232
Contraception. *See also* Oral
  contraceptives
    barrier methods, 183
    clip sterilization, 184

    low-dose birth-control pills, 183–84
    during menopause, 181
    new copper IUD, 183
    sterilization, 184
Cooking utensils, iron, 125
Cool, Creamy Dressing, 116
Cool and Fruity Dessert, 82
Copper deficiency, sleep and, 10
Corn oil, 58
Cramps, muscle, 288–89
Cravings, weight-loss and, 100
Creativity, middle age and, 189
Crossed eyes, 224–25
CTS. *See* Carpal tunnel syndrome
Cycling, backache and, 266, 283–84

D
Dairy products, hypertension and, 81
Deep-breathing exercises, 277
Dehydration, chills and, 297–98
Deodorant, allergy reactions and, 269
Depression, 6, 152–53
Dessert, calories in, 176
Diabetes
    high-mono diet and, 14
    magnesium and, 146–47
    nopal cactus and, 161
Diaphragm, spasms in, 292
Diet pills, hypertension and, 170
Digestive problems
    belching, 299
    diverticula, 304
    flatulence, 300–302
    gas, 299–302
    heartburn, 302–4
    hemorrhoids, 304–5
    irritable bowel syndrome, 303–4
    preparing beans to avoid, 301
Diuretics, magnesium and, 146
Diuril, magnesium and, 146
Diverticula, 304
Drug(s)
    anticancer, 160–61
    antihypertensive, 172
    for lowering high cholesterol, 221–22
    vitamin B_6 and, 154
Dry socket, vitamin C and, 16
Ductwork, indoor air pollution and, 192–93

E
Ear piercing
    AIDS virus and, 199
    allergy reactions and, 268

Ears, swimming and, 292
Eating, healing and, 75–76
Elbows, pain in, 292–93
Employment, middle age and, 188
Energy-efficient homes, indoor air pollution and, 196–97
Estrogen, vitamin B$_6$ and, 155
Exercise
    aging and, 179, 181
    bones and, 165
    cancer-fighting benefit of, 19
    cardiovascular system and, 181
    deep-breathing, TMJ disorders and, 277
    easy, weight loss and, 102–3
    high-density lipoprotein and, 221
    hypertension and, 83
    Kegel, 185
    postoperative recovery and, 203–5
    prevention of depression and, 6
    progressive relaxation, TMJ disorders and, 277
    vitamin E and, 21
    weight loss and, 96–97, 108–9
    with weights, 177
Eye exercises. *See* Vision therapy
Eyes
    redness of, 286
    sunburn of, 286–87
    vision therapy for, 224–25

F
Facial care
    cleansing, 307–9
    rinsing, 309
    toning, 309–10
Family members, hypertension and, 172
Fast foods, hypertension and, 170–71
Fat(s)
    breast cancer and, 88–89, 90
    calories in, 176
    counting grams of, 93
    cravings for, weight loss and, 119–21
    hypertension and, 167
    monounsaturated, 14, 36–40
    polyunsaturated, differences in, 50
    reducing intake of, 92
Feet, chilled, 295
Feverfew, 159–60
Fiber, 22–23
    cancer and, 55
    cholesterol and, 62–63
    insoluble, 23

iron absorption and, 125
    soluble, 23–24
    sources of, 25
    supplemental, 26, 28
Fiber-rich diet, 24–28, 46
Fibrositis, 206
Figs, dried, 58
Fish, hypertension and, 80, 166, 169
Fish oil, 49. *See also* Omega-3 fats
    arthritis and, 71–72
    heart and, 51
    hypertension and, 166
    late asthma reaction and, 17
    rheumatoid arthritis and, 2
    supplemental, 53
Flatulence, 300–302
Flexibility, 177, 179
Flexural dermatitis, 290
Fluids, healing and, 76
Folate, 8
Folk cures, 159
Food(s). *See specific foods;* Fast foods, hypertension and
    anticancer, 45, 54–61
    hot, chills and, 297
    iron-fortified, 126
    "no cholesterol," 217
    nutritionist's choices of, 44–49
Formaldehyde
    allergy reactions and, 269
    indoor air pollution and, 195–96
Fruit, hypertension and, 81–82
Fungi
    garlic and, 74
    mutant, anticancer drugs and, 160–61
Furnace(s), indoor air pollution and, 192–95
Furosemide, magnesium and, 146

G
Garlic, 72–75
Ginkgo extracts, 162
Glucose levels, 14
Glutamate, 149
Glycine, muscles and, 150–52
Golf, backache and, 284
Grafts, skin, vitamin E and, 141
Grapefruit, 58
Great northern beans, 58
Greens, collard, 58
Guided imagery, 277

H
Hair dye, allergy reactions and, 269
Hands, chilled, 295
HDL. *See* High-density lipoprotein

Headaches, exercise-induced, 287
Healing 75–76, 160
Heart
    omega-3 fats and, 50–51
    walking and, 228–29
Heart attack, magnesium and, 145
Heartburn, 302–3
Heart disease, HDL and risk for, 20
Heat, TMJ disorders and, 274–75
Heat exhaustion, 287–88
Hemorrhoids, 304–5
High blood pressure. *See*
Hypertension
High-Calcium Stir-Fry, 80
High-density lipoprotein (HDL)
    alcohol and, 221
    exercise and, 221
    levels of heart disease and, 20
    walking and, 229–30
High-Fiber Oat Bread, 27
Hobbies, weight loss and, 96
Homosexuality, AIDS virus and, 201
Honey, unprocessed, 160
Honey/Berry Frozen Yogurt
    Pops, 84
Hormone-replacement therapy
    (HRT), 185, 187
Hot flashes, 187. *See also*
    Menopause
HRT. *See* Hormone-replacement
    therapy
Hummus, 118
Humor, weight loss and, 97
Hydralazine, 154
Hypertension, 77–78. *See also* Blood
    pressure
    alcoholic beverages and, 79, 167
    anger and, 171
    baked potatoes and, 168
    calcium and, 79
    calmness and, 172
    chewing tobacco and, 173
    cigarette smoking and, 172
    cooking vegetables and, 168
    dietary sodium and, 169–70
    diet pills and, 170
    drinking water and, 170
    exercise and, 83
    family members and, 172
    fast foods and, 170–71
    fats and, 167
    fish and, 80, 166
    fish oil and, 166
    fruit and, 81–82
    "hidden" salt and, 171
    laughing and, 170
    low-fat dairy products and, 81

    magnesium and, 145–46
    medication for, 172
    muscle relaxation and, 171
    music and, 172
    nondrug approaches to, 78–87
    oral contraceptives and, 168
    petting animals and, 168–69
    potatoes and, 82–83
    recipes for reducing, 80, 82, 83,
        84, 85
    relaxation and, 83
    salt and, 80–81, 169–70
    scents and, 171
    snack foods and, 84
    soft water and, 167
    stress and, 169
    talking to self and, 172
    vegetables and, 85
    walking and, 78, 80, 81, 166–67
    watching fish in aquariums and,
        169
    weight and, 166
    "white-coat," 167
    yogurt and, 84

I
IBS. *See* Irritable bowel syndrome
Imagery, interactive, 255–56
Immunity
    vitamin B_6 and, 157
    vitamin E and, 140
Infants, massage and, 5
Inflexibility, 177, 179
Influenza, garlic and, 74–75
Insomnia, 205–6. *See also* Sleep
Intelligence, middle age and, 189–90
Intelligence quotient. *See* IQ
Interactive imagery, 255–56
Intermittent claudication, 288
IQ, 256–57
Iron
    absorption of
        calcium and, 124
        coffee and, 125
        fiber and, 125
        tea and, 125
        vitamin C and, 125
    in beans, 124–25
    cooking utensils, 125
    deficiency of
        chills and, 294–95
        sleep and, 10
    in meats, 123–24
    in peas, 124–25
    supplemental, 126
    in vegetables, 124
Iron-deficiency anemia, 122–27

Iron-fortified foods, 126
Irritable bowel syndrome (IBS),
    303–4
Isoleucine, 149
Isoniazid, 154

K
Kale, 58
Kegel exercise, sex life and, 185
Kerosene heaters, indoor air
    pollution and, 194
Kidney beans, 58–59
Kidney stones, vitamin B₆ and, 155
Kissing, AIDS virus and, 199
Kiwifruit, 59
Knees, pain in, 290–91

L
Lasix, magnesium and, 146
Laughter, hypertension and, 170
Lazy eyes, vision therapy for, 225
LDL. *See* Low-density lipoprotein,
    monounsaturated fat and
Leucine, 149
Life, mission in, 243–44
    work and, 246–47
Lovastatin, 222
Low-density lipoprotein (LDL),
    monounsaturated fat and, 38
Low-fat diet, 46, 52–53
    breast cancer and, 87–91
    cancer and, 55
L-phenylalanine, 152–53
Lubrin, 185
Lung cancer, beta-carotene and, 129
Lungs, B vitamins and, 8

M
Magnesium, 143, 147–48
    arrhythmias and, 143–44
    cancer and, 146
    cholesterol levels and, 144–45
    diabetes and, 146–47
    diuretics and, 146
    heart attack and, 145
    high blood pressure and, 145–46
    pregnancy and, 147
    sources of, 148
    symptoms of deficiency of, 143
Malaria, Chinese treatment for, 161
Mangoes, 59
Marital burnout, 187
Marriage, middle age and, 187–88
Massage, infants and, 5
Meat(s)
    iron in, 123–24
    protein in, 164

Medicine, future for, 259–60
Memory, 252–53
    interactive imagery and, 255–56
    lapses in, middle age and,
        189–90
    memorizing and, 253–54
    observation and, 254
Menopause
    birth control and, 181, 183–84
    help for, 187
Metabolic rate
    aging and, 181
    slowdown of, 176
Mevacor, 222
Middle age, 173
    birth control and, 181, 183–84
    body conditioning for, 177–81
    boredom and, 187
    brainpower and, 189–90
    cardiovascular conditioning for,
        181
    contraception for, 181–84
    creativity and, 189
    employment and, 188
    healthy relationships for, 187–88
    intelligence and, 189–90
    job transition for, 188
    makeovers, 175, 178, 180,
        182–83, 186
    marital burnout and, 187
    marriage and, 187–88
    memory lapses and, 189–90
    menopause and, 187
    metabolic slowdown in, 176
    nutrition for, 173–77
    sex and, 184–85, 187
Middle-age spread, 179
Migraine headaches, feverfew and,
    159–60
Milk, skim, 60
    evaporated, 58
Mineral(s). *See also specific types*
    aging and, 173–74
    coffee and, 174
    deficiency of, sleep problems
        and, 10
    tea and, 174
Minilaparotomy, 184
Moduretic, magnesium and, 146
Monounsaturated fat, 38–40
    diabetes and, 14
    heart and, 36–38
    sources of, 40
    studies on, 36–38
Motivation, weight loss and, 101–2,
    109
Multivitamins, preconception, 18

Muscle(s)
 amino acids and, 150–52
 conditioning of, 177
 cramps, 288–89
 relaxation, hypertension and,
  171
 strains, 289
  rebound tactics for, 11
Music, hypertension and, 172
Mutant fungi, anticancer drugs and,
 160–61
Myopia, 224–25

N
Nail polish, allergy reactions and,
 268
Napping, 208–9. *See also* Sleep
Nearsightedness, 224–25
Nibbler's Weight-Loss Plan, 113–16
 recipes for, 116–19
Nine-Bean Soup, 68
Nonsmokers' etiquette, 210–16
Nopal cactus, diabetes and, 161
Nordic ski machine, for backache,
 266
Nutrition, 44–49
Nuts, Brazil, 56

O
Oat bran
 cholesterol and, 62–63
 recipes for, 67
Oat Bran-Raisin Muffins, 67
Oatmeal, 59
Obesity, osteoarthritis and, 15. *See
 also* Weight loss
Observation, memory and, 254
Occlusive folliculitis, 284
Occupation, personal meaning of,
 241–43
Oil(s), 58
Olive oil, 38–40
Omega-3 fats, 49, 218. *See also* Fish
 oil
 cancer and, 52
 heart and, 50–51
Omega-6 fats, 50
Oral contraceptives. *See also*
 Contraception
 hypertension and, 168
 low-dose, 183–84
Oranges, 59
Ornithine, muscles and, 151
Osteoarthritis
 description of, 69–70
 diet and, 70
 obesity and, 15

Osteoporosis, candidates for, 162–65
Oxylate, calcium absorption and, 164

P
Papaya, 59
Parkinson's disease, 137–39
Peas 59, 124–25
Penicillamine, 154
Peppers, sweet, 60
Pets, 168–69, 200
Phosphate, calcium and, 163–64
Plateaus, in weight loss, 103
Pollution. *See* Air pollution, indoor
Polyunsaturated fats, 50
Popcorn, 59
Postoperative recovery, 203–5
Posture, TMJ disorders and, 275–76
Potatoes
 as anticancer food, 59
 hypertension and, 82–83, 168
 sweet, 61
PR. *See* Progressive relaxation
Pregnancy, magnesium and, 147
Primrose oil, 2
Progressive relaxation (PR)
 power of, 249–51
 successful, 251–52
 TMJ disorders and, 277
Propranolol, hypertension and, 172
Protein, 41, 43–44
 amyotrophic lateral sclerosis
  and, 149–50
 excess, 164
 myths about, 41–43
Prunes, 59–60
Pumpkin, 60
Pyridoxal, 157–58
Pyridoxamine, 157–58
Pyridoxine, 157–58

Q
Questran, 222

R
Racquetball, backache and, 267
Radon, indoor air pollution and, 196
Raisins, 60
Rapeseed oil, 58
Rashes, 289–90
Rational thinking, 257–58
Raynaud's syndrome, 298–99
Relationships, walking and, 231–32
Relaxation. *See also* Progressive
 relaxation (PR)
 hypertension and, 83, 171
 TMJ disorders and, 277
Renal calculus, vitamin B_6 and, 155

Rheumatoid arthritis, 2
Rice, brown, 57
Roughage. *See* Fiber
Rowing machine, backache and, 266
Runner's knee, 290–91
Running, backache and, 267
Rutabagas, 61

S
Saddle sores, 291
Salmon, canned, 60
Salt. *See* Sodium, dietary
Sardines, canned, 60
Scents, hypertension and, 171
Seizures, vitamin B₆ and, 157
Selenium, cancer and, 55–56, 131
Sex
    AIDS virus and, 201, 202–3
    Kegel exercises and, 185
    middle age and, 184–85, 187
    sleep and, 207
    swimming and, 13
Shoulder tendinitis, 291–92
Side stitches, 292
Skim milk, 60
    evaporated, 58
Skin
    around the eyes, 280–81
    knowledge about, 279–80
    moisturizing of, 281–82
    vitamin E and, 141
Sleep. *See also* Insomnia
    age and, 206
    anxiety and, 207
    deprivation of, 206–7
        chronic, 207–8
    executives and, 206
    lack of, 207
    mineral deficiencies and, 10
    napping, 208–9
    necessary amount of, 205–6
    sex and, 207
Sleep positions, 209
    night bruxism and, 7
    teeth grinding and, 7
Smoking. *See* Cigarette smoking
Snack foods, hypertension and, 84
Snacking, weight loss and, 110–12
    evening, 116
    midafternoon, 114–15
    midmorning, 113–14
    plan for, 113–16
    recipes for, 116–19
Snake venom, blood clots and, 1
Sodium, dietary
    hidden, 171

    hypertension and, 80–81, 169–70
    in water, 170
Soft drinks, phosphate in, 163–64
Spinach, 60
Spironolactone, magnesium and, 146
Sprains, 292
Squash, butternut, 57
Starch, 28
Strabismus, visual therapy for,
    224–25
Strains, muscle, 289
Strawberries, 60
Stress
    chills and, 297
    hypertension and, 169
    immediate, 248–49
    long-term, 248–49
    TMJ disorders and, 276–77
Stroke, snake venom and, 1
Sunburn, to eyes, 286–87
Sunflower seeds, 60
Sweet or Savory Yogurt Cheese, 117
Sweet peppers, 60
Sweet potatoes, 61
Swimmer's ear, 292
Swimming
    AIDS virus and, 198–99
    backache and, 266, 283–84
    eye redness and, 286
    sex and, 13
Swordfish, 61

T
Table salt. *See* Sodium, dietary
Tannins, in coffee and tea, 174
Tea, 174–75
    iron absorption and, 125
Teeth grinding, 7
Television, 189
Temporomandibular joint disorders.
    See TMJ disorders
Tendinitis, shoulder, 291
Tendons, conditioning of, 177
Tennis, backache and, 267, 284
Tennis elbow, 292–93
Tennis toe, 293
Tension, 248
Theophylline, vitamin B₆ deficiency
    and, 154
Thermogenesis, 297
Thinking, rational, 257–59
Three-Bean Salad, 85
TMJ disorders, 270–72
    bad posture and, 275–76
    caffeine and, 274
    cold application for, 274–75